Lost

Critical Issues in Health and Medicine

Edited by Rima D. Apple, University of Wisconsin–Madison, and Janet Golden, Rutgers University, Camden

Growing criticism of the U.S. health care system is coming from consumers, politicians, the media, activists, and health care professionals. Critical Issues in Health and Medicine is a collection of books that explores these contemporary dilemmas from a variety of perspectives, among them political, legal, historical, sociological, and comparative, and with attention to crucial dimensions such as race, gender, ethnicity, sexuality, and culture.

For a list of titles in the series, see the last page of the book.

Lost

~

Miscarriage in Nineteenth-Century America

SHANNON WITHYCOMBE

Rutgers University Press

New Brunswick, Camden, and Newark, New Jersey, and London

Names: Withycombe, Shannon, author.
Title: Lost : miscarriage in nineteenth-century America / Shannon Withycombe.
Description: New Brunswick : Rutgers University Press, [2018] | Includes
bibliographical references and index.
Identifiers: LCCN 2017059908| ISBN 9780813591544 (cloth : alk. paper) |
ISBN 9780813591537 (pbk. : alk. paper) | ISBN 9780813591551 (epub) |
ISBN 9780813591575 (pdf)
Subjects: | MESH: Abortion, Spontaneous—history | Abortion,
Spontaneous—psychology | Pregnancy—psychology | Fetal Research—history |
History, 19th Century | United States
Classification: LCC RG648 | NLM WQ 11 AA1 | DDC 618.3/92—dc23
LC record available at https://lccn.loc.gov/2017059908

A British Cataloging-in-Publication record for this book is available
from the British Library.

∞ The paper used in this publication meets the requirements of the American
National Standard for Information Sciences—Permanence of Paper for Printed
Library Materials, ANSI Z39.48-1992.

www.rutgersuniversitypress.org

Manufactured in the United States of America

For all the women who have lost

Contents

Lost

Introduction

When the poet Henry Wadsworth Longfellow decided to take his wife, Mary, on an extended trip through Europe in 1835, Mary asked her childhood friend, Clara Crowninshield, to come along as her companion. For the next year, Crowninshield kept a daily diary, noting the unique characters, breathtaking sights, flirtations, and tragedies with which she met while in Europe. On the night of October 5, 1835, while in Amsterdam, Crowninshield awoke to a tap at her door. Longfellow was looking for a candle, as his had burned down while he stayed up, watching over his ill wife. Crowninshield described the encounter: "'Is anything the matter,' said I. 'Yes' said he, 'Mary is sick—worse than ever.'" Crowninshield remained in her room until morning when she asked Longfellow if Mary had had an ague fit. "Something worse than that," he had replied.[1]

In his own journal, Longfellow described the event as well: "Was up before daylight—Mary being very ill. . . . Sent for the Dr. in a hurry; but before he arrived it was all over."[2] Mary rallied, and the party moved on to Rotterdam, but her health soon took a turn for the worse. On November 28, Longfellow wrote to his father: "I am very much grieved to say, that Mary is not so well to-day. She is extremely feeble; and the physicians tell me that her situation is dangerous. It is the effect of a miscarriage, which happened some weeks ago, in spite of all our precautions . . . God grant that she may recover; —but if this is not his will, may we all be resigned to whatever he may ordain."[3] Mary Longfellow died the following day.

This account of a pregnancy loss, one that includes illness, death, and sorrow, is what I expected of miscarriage in the nineteenth century when I began this research. As an event frequently described in modern terms as a tragedy, something requiring emotional recovery, a trauma causing grief and depression, or as something to cope with, it makes sense that miscarriage would have been even more difficult, sadder, and deadlier two centuries ago.[4] Mary Longfellow's travails fit neatly within the historical narrative of the nineteenth-century woman being a slave to reproduction, and in danger of losing her life to it. Certainly, the writings of Crowninshield and Longfellow prove that narrative could be appropriate, but this book will reveal that the reality of nineteenth-century miscarriage in the United States was constructed from multiple narratives. This book provides a history of miscarriage that does not presuppose loss, tragedy, or failure. Instead, I want to investigate pregnancy loss without any assumption of how the various actors involved might have felt or acted at the time. A detailed analysis of women's personal writings about the phenomenon, as well as stories gleaned from medical reports and hospital records, unveil representations of pregnancy loss that in fact show that nineteenth-century miscarriage was so much more complex than the one tragic story of Mary Longfellow.[5]

Lost demonstrates how women experienced miscarriage in a world without early pregnancy tests, ultrasounds, or legal reproductive control. In the process, it reveals how Americans interpreted, and continue to interpret, miscarriage within a complex web of reproductive desires, expectations, and abilities. This book utilizes women's own writings about miscarriage for the first time to explore individual understandings of pregnancy loss and the multiple social and medical forces that helped to shape those perceptions. When I embarked on this research in graduate school, a senior scholar asked, somewhat dubiously, "Will you be able to find these sources?" I admit I was dubious, as well, but doggedly determined. I had no interest in telling the history of miscarriage without the inclusion of women's voices. The story of miscarriage gleaned only from published medical sources could provide some understanding of how the event fit into a medical history of reproduction, or how physicians used the event to increase business and authority over American childbearing. But gaining access to how women discussed the experience—with loved ones through letters and with themselves in private diaries—would allow me to better understand the lived experience and personal interpretations of miscarriage in nineteenth-century America.

To be sure, finding these private discussions was not easy. I spent years sifting through collections of family papers, searching for conversations I thought would prove fruitful, such as the five years of correspondence between Blanche Butler Ames and her husband, Adelbert. Upon finding such potentially rich collections, I then figured out which months and years were most likely to contain a mention of a miscarriage based on the birth of live children. Miscarriages do not tend to show up on family trees or in finding aids, and so I spent many, many hours reading through letters and journals searching for some clue that a woman might have lost a pregnancy. Some of my most exciting days in the archives were when I found a woman describing knitting "tiny socks" or the arrival of a "little stranger" to a loved one when I knew she had had no live births that year. In the end, these long hours were well spent, for they resulted not only in personal descriptions of miscarriage, but also the rich detail of these women's lives—the daily struggles, the family tensions, and the interpersonal relationships—that helped me better contextualize their reactions to a pregnancy loss. Only by immersing myself in the lives and words of these women could I properly understand the complexity of this bodily and reproductive event.

While miscarrying women hold center stage in this book, I am also interested, as a historian of medicine, in the role of doctors in miscarriage at the time. Published medical writings on miscarriage were certainly much easier to find, but I still strive to contextualize each published report, teaching textbook, and medical lecture. I have no interest in portraying victims or villains or in describing a homogenous group of practitioners following some predetermined script. Instead, I strive to consider each case of miscarriage individually—Who was there? Why were they there? What happened? Why did it happen that way? I make no assumptions about the power of regular physicians had over their patients, or vice versa. Instead, I use these cases to expose the tricky negotiations carried out in the midst of a bloody and painful event.

Weaving together women's personal writings and doctors' publications from 1820 to 1912, *Lost* investigates the transformative changes that took place in how Americans conceptualized pregnancy, understood miscarriage, and interpreted fetal tissues over the course of the nineteenth century. This juxtaposition of women and doctors creates a narrative that takes us from the early nineteenth century, when doctors frequently interpreted miscarriage materials as foreign fruits or nonhuman objects, to the dawn of professional embryology at the turn of the twentieth century, when physicians viewed these materials as valuable for scientific research. It also follows the transformation of the corporeality of miscarriage and its understanding, from a situation "known" by women who experienced its inner turmoil, to an event "known" by doctors who entered the female body and gained a view that was inaccessible to their patients.

Scholars have long contended that pregnancy and miscarriage interpretations are firmly tied to women's social roles.[6] In nineteenth-century America, when women's primary role was the bearing and rearing of children, I initially assumed that miscarriage would be considered a failure or a shameful event. Instead, I found individual women who described the experience openly, without reference to shame or failure, and some who even expressed outright joy at the event. Focusing on miscarriage exposes the fragility of narratives that depict static social roles based merely on gender.

As we can see from the case of Mary Longfellow, miscarriage was not an activity that all women experienced alone or only with female companions. Families frequently relied on male doctors to attend to miscarriage cases in larger numbers than they would for childbirth during the same period.[7] A miscarriage carried markers of a medical emergency—it produced bleeding, pain, fever, and perhaps most importantly, it was an example of a natural procedure (pregnancy and birth) going wrong. Although early in the nineteenth century many of the women relying on medical attention to help them through miscarriage were wealthy, by the 1870s doctors attended miscarriage cases in tenement buildings, charity hospitals, and homes of the poor. While *Lost* shows that social and personal circumstances greatly shaped how women understood and responded to their miscarriages, it also exposes the growing interest in including physicians in the experience.

One goal of this book is to insert miscarriage into the history of reproduction and fertility, bringing it to a wider audience.[8] At the same time, I want to show how the inclusion of pregnancy loss into the history of American women and reproduction changes our understanding of the medicalization of the female body. The current literature on the medicalization of reproduction is rich, and it includes studies on childbirth, birth control, abortion, infertility, and menopause.[9] Miscarriage at once fits within these existing narratives, and yet it shows distinct differences in the motivation of the medical practitioners involved. A common narrative claims that the efforts of regular doctors to gain a monopoly over the marketplace, help stem the rising tide of infant and maternal mortality, and respond to consumer demand were all reasons for this increase in the medical oversight of American reproduction between the nineteenth and twentieth centuries. But what a study on miscarriage also reveals is the desire of physicians to incorporate science as a legitimizing force in their medical practices. The medicalization of miscarriage was, at least in part, a result of doctors' eagerness to secure the products of miscarriage—unique scientific specimens. Some of the impetus for doctors to rush to the bedsides of pregnant and birthing women was that they might have a chance to obtain these tiny specimens—objects portable enough to put in one's pocket and yet magnificent beings that could expose a wealth of information about human biology. A movement that led eventually to the establishment of the internationally renowned Carnegie Institute Department of Embryology, and what later became known as the "great embryo hunt," began among everyday general practitioners who understood the value of these small tissues—both in terms of what could be learned from them, and of their value as professional markers.[10]

In addition, this book forces us to rethink our conception of late nineteenth-century American reproduction. Commonly, this era is described in terms of restrictions—both in what was available to women as means to control their fertility, and in terms of women's social roles. In the latter half of the century, women looked to restrict their childbearing (as proven by the falling birth rate), but they faced a society that both tamped down on their ability to do so (with the illegalization of birth control and abortion) and informed them that they should look to mothering as their only occupation and lifestyle. It could be too easy to assume that women living in this time found little in the way of acceptance of their reproductive failures. If a woman's primary role was to have children, then failing at a pregnancy could mean she had failed in her role as a woman. And yet, *Lost* shows that nineteenth-century women found a free space to think of their miscarriages in terms that suited their personal, familial, economic, and religious lives, a space carved out by those very restrictions. The reality of women's lives—trying to have fewer children and having no reliable way to do so—created a social world in which miscarriage was not a failure of motherhood, the products of miscarriage were not children or infants, and doctors could freely take fetal tissues away for scientific study and display.

This book uncovers how, over the course of the nineteenth century, as restrictions upon women's fertility increased, many women fought back, crafting meanings of their miscarriages that made sense and felt comfortable. At the same time, women's experiences of pregnancy and miscarriage, and their desire to limit their families, shaped twentieth-century embryology. Doctors could only obtain their large collections of fetal tissues with the help of their female patients, patients who were perhaps eager to see their miscarriages as producing specimens rather than children. For many women, pregnancy did not make a child—birthing did. Therefore, they could freely hand over tissues without feelings of guilt, or social repercussions. Women's desires to find solace in miscarriage shaped the corporeal limits of motherhood. A woman could sense she was pregnant, feel motion within her uterus, and yet still never call herself a mother if the pregnancy failed. Without a child, she was not yet a mother. This corporeal boundary of motherhood aided doctors who were seeking the desired tissues. They could navigate this tricky enterprise—using the products of reproduction to further scientific study without appearing to profit from the death of children—because many women sought the result that miscarriage brought: smaller families.

A history of miscarriage may begin with questions of how many, how often, and how did it affect women? But, as this book shows, that is not where it ends. A history of miscarriage entails questions of bodily expertise, family desires, corporeality, and the benefits of ambiguity. Throughout the nineteenth century, two major shifts took place in American miscarriage, both of which altered the corporeality of the experience. In the first few decades of the nineteenth century, pregnancy and miscarriage were phenomena felt internally by women while doctors could determine these states only externally. Women's initial lack of faith in medical attention for miscarriage was due in part to this corporeal separation. By the 1870s, however, doctors claimed that only by entering the body, through the vaginal canal and into the uterus, could one truly understand a miscarriage. At the same time, this line of reasoning promoted a view of the body that was unavailable to their female patients, thus shifting the focus to a medical construction of miscarriage.

Doctors and women also worked to alter the bodies produced by miscarriage during this time. Although these products of miscarriage were initially viewed as foreign fruits or bloody masses of little scientific value, physicians redefined these objects, in the decades following the rise in popularity of epigenesis and the emergence of embryology, into important tools for the study of human development. Fetal bodies gained new value by virtue of their perceived rarity and their perceived utility to science. By the 1880s, doctors interpreted these new scientific specimens as indubitably human, and thus as vital representations of both humanity and life.

While surveying the published medical literature on miscarriage can reveal the collective "women" imagined by regular doctors, such a collective does not exist in reality. This book strives to capture the variety and richness of nineteenth-century American women's experiences with miscarriage, giving voice to wealthy, middling, and working-class poor white women, poor European immigrant women, unmarried and married women, and free African American women. This book does not include all groups of women living in the United States from 1820 to 1912, however. It leaves out, for example, native women, eastern European immigrant women, and enslaved women. Rather than attempting to access all women's experiences (admittedly an impossible task), *Lost* focuses on a close analysis of individual women. Responding to a miscarriage, or making meaning of its material results, was a complex decision-making process, and we need to understand many facets of a woman's life before comprehending why she expressed joy, sorrow, or indifference to her miscarriage. Utilizing large collections of correspondence and diaries can expose how particular women thought about pregnancy, motherhood, their role in their family and their community, and how all these aspects shaped their interpretations of miscarriage. This close analysis, while certainly leaving out some viewpoints, allows us to better understand the forces at work in all women's miscarriage experiences.

The book complements individual stories with glimpses of women who left fewer documents behind. Hospital records from the New England Hospital for Women and Children, a charity hospital serving unmarried and poor women of Boston, allow us entry into the world of working women, and single women whose miscarriages might have been especially welcomed. Doctors' case reports shed light on the experiences of working-class women in other cities, as well as those of free African American women. Accessing these stories allows us to better analyze the particular narratives provided and to determine to what extent forces such as race and class shaped miscarriage interpretations and realities.

The book is framed primarily around the social and medical shifts at work in the middle of the nineteenth century. At that time doctors began to rally for their place at the bedside of miscarrying women, which coincided with an increased public effort to restrict women's access to fertility control. Chapter 1 explores the individual miscarriage experiences of four women in the nineteenth century as a way to understand how miscarriage is deeply intertwined in a complex web of family, economics, geography, personal desires, and faith in medicine. As fertility rates plummeted in the late nineteenth century, but restrictions against fertility control increased, women found themselves desiring smaller families but with little in the way of safe or effective means to accomplish this. Within this context, some women understood miscarriage to be a happy event or a welcomed relief. Only when we understand the reproductive desires and realities facing women at the time can we truly grasp the individual, medical, and social constructions of pregnancy loss.

Chapter 2 investigates the earlier history of miscarriage in the eighteenth and early nineteenth century and explores the development of embryology and the philosophical debates about human creation that altered how many Americans understood pregnancy. Prior to 1800, miscarriage was a condition that was often diagnosed only after the expelled product could be proven to be a normally developing infant. Since most early-term miscarriages do not produce objects easily recognized as human infants, many doctors and women in the Western world described "false" pregnancies and conceptualized the pregnant condition as one rife with ambiguity. As German scholars began to develop the science of embryology, American doctors reevaluated miscarriage and began to see it as a medical puzzle, rather than merely as a family issue.

Chapter 3 examines physicians' initial attempts to redefine miscarriage as a medical issue, and how those first attempts at medicalization largely failed. By the 1840s, doctors viewed miscarriage as something about which they should have some expertise. What they previously viewed as nature's fix to a pregnancy gone wrong they now constructed as nature's mistake that required a medical solution. By examining popular domestic health guides and women's personal writings alongside the more professional writings of physicians, however, we can see that doctors actually had little to offer to potential patients. Initially focusing on miscarriage causes, physicians presented women with long lists that served more to sustain the view that miscarriage was unavoidable, leaving many women unconvinced that medical aid could help prevent a pregnancy loss. After the 1860s, doctors gained access to many miscarriage cases due to social and economic shifts, and, as illustrated in Chapter 4, they began incorporating aggressive and intrusive treatment into their miscarriage responses. However, as I contend throughout the book, this transformation in medical practice was not a movement of doctors alone, but it was also a response of many women who benefited from this new medical attention. As women moved away from their extended families and familiar communities because of industrialization and urbanization in the second half of the nineteenth century, they looked to doctors for help in miscarriage cases in unprecedented numbers, and their desires for action, results, and reproductive control helped to shape emerging medical expertise in pregnancy loss.

The final chapter focuses on the material products of miscarriage. Chapter 5 demonstrates that doctors sought the medicalization of miscarriage not only for the increase in practice and prestige, but also for the valuable scientific specimens they could obtain at the bedside. But physicians needed the cooperation of miscarrying women, their families, and sometimes their female attendants. Together, professional physicians and lay women shaped the emerging scientific field of human embryology. Regular physicians conducted scientific research on fetal and placental tissues that emerged though miscarriage, but they did so only at the behest of families that invited doctors to attend pregnancy-loss cases and handed over the resulting tissues.

This book revolves around the ambiguities of nineteenth-century pregnancy, miscarriage, and the bodies involved in these processes, and some of this ambiguity necessarily involves an ambiguity of language, indicating the limits of language with respect to these new objects. In nineteenth-century America (and up through much of the twentieth century as well) the words "abortion" and "miscarriage" were virtually interchangeable. Women wrote of an "abortion" in a way that makes it clear that the event was neither intended nor induced, while doctors described "abortions" with a variety of causes, most being accidental. Another point of potential confusion is the usage of "fetus," "ovum," and "embryo." These terms were primarily used by medical writers, but often with no discernable pattern. In his 1866 publication, Chicago physician Edwin Hale provided a helpful division of miscarriage based on the objects involved: "(1) Ovular, when the ovum is lost before it is impregnated. (2) Embryonic, when the impregnated ovum is expelled before the placenta has formed its uterine attachment. (3) Foetal, when the expulsion occurs after the last date, and before the viability of the child."[11] Other doctors followed Hale's divisions in describing the product of a miscarriage in these three sequential terms, but just as many used the terms indiscriminately, with no obvious reference to age or placental attachment.[12] In this book, when referring to a historical source, I will use the terms of the writer (fetus, embryo, abortion). In my own analysis, I will rely upon the familiar term "miscarriage" to refer to an accidental pregnancy loss. In discussing the tissues involved, I will use the somewhat clunky but neutral terms "products of miscarriage" or "fetal tissues" to avoid anachronistic judgments of what historical actors saw in various cases—a blood clot, a small body, or a child.

Even if the term "abortion" in the nineteenth century carried a meaning different from the meaning used today, medical writers often defined it, and thus we gain some understanding of what they meant. Terms like "fetus," however, remain far murkier. A word like "fetus" has no firm basis in an objective reality. It has meant different things to different people, and it has been far from a stable concept over time. Exactly what a doctor was remembering or imagining when writing about a "fetus" is not something we can know with much precision. In some instances, we can find images or graphic descriptions of the tissues and bodies involved, but we cannot assume parity between what a doctor in 1875 described as a fetus and the modern image of a fetus as it appears in an ultrasound. We must remember that in this era of intense transformation of reproductive realities, embryological studies, and medical authority, there may not have been the language available to accurately describe what doctors or their patients saw, felt, and experienced.

In placing a bodily event at the center of my study, this book expands and challenges multiple fields of scholarship. By detailing the fetal and placental tissues expelled by miscarrying women and avidly studied and shared by physicians, I push the history of embryology beyond the boundaries of laboratories, male elites, and professional science. A deep analysis of women's descriptions of their pregnant and miscarrying bodies exposes the restrictions of recent scholarship linking modern visualization technologies and understandings of "the unborn" within American pregnancy. Finally, unearthing nineteenth-century women's reflections on their own miscarriages questions academic, activist, and medical work that assumes a universal response of grief in all cases of pregnancy loss.

As scholars have noted in recent years, our current culture has constructed a wall of silence surrounding the topic of miscarriage.[13] Women find themselves unsure of how to talk about the experience, wondering if it is proper to announce it to family or coworkers, and they are caught in a web of confusion about their emotions in the wake of the phenomenon. More than one colleague has remarked to me, upon learning of my research, that they had no idea how prevalent miscarriage was until they, or their partner, had their own. Experts estimate that 15–30 percent of all pregnancies end in miscarriage—a statistic that birthing guides or classes rarely share with pregnant women.[14] As part of the recent call to break the silence about pregnancy loss, *Lost* brings to light how women of the past understood this bodily and family event, and this historical context gives us a new perspective on our own practices as well as a model for moving beyond our current restrictive and secretive miscarriage culture.

1

Oh Joy, Oh Rapture

Describing the Nineteenth-Century Miscarriage

In 1875, Emily FitzGerald suffered a miscarriage. That same year, Annie Van Ness lost her first pregnancy. In 1879, Mary Cheney wrote a letter to her husband with news of the failure of her latest pregnancy. Reading these statements in the twenty-first century evokes sadness, but also familiarity. We live in a world where celebrities reveal their own struggles with pregnancy loss, and physicians conduct scientific studies exposing the guilt and shame felt by families dealing with miscarriage.[1] We are used to imagining miscarrying women as coping, damaged, failing, and sad.

And yet, the three sentences I wrote to open this chapter are patently false. That is not what happened in nineteenth-century America. Although each woman did miscarry a pregnancy, according to their own words their experiences had nothing to do with suffering, loss, or failure. A look into the history of miscarriage, and into how women described the experience themselves, reveals that interpretations of miscarriage in terms of loss or tragedy are modern constructs, not ahistorical meanings somehow inherent to the experience. Emily FitzGerald, Annie Van Ness, and Mary Cheney instead described their experiences in terms of comfort and relief, and they even used words like "joy."

Personal writings of women living and miscarrying in the nineteenth century expose the range and fluidity of responses in how women of that time understood what or who resided and grew within their expanding bodies. As a modern reader, I was continually surprised that these letters and diary entries contained such a variety of reactions, emotions, and responses to miscarriage. I had learned from my graduate education that the late nineteenth century was marked by two phenomena that should have shaped miscarriage in particular ways—the narrowing of the definition of femininity and the development of embryology. As women began to step outside of the home for employment, higher education, and even political activism toward the close of the century, physicians, popular periodicals, and public officials reacted by discussing the biological and innate link between femininity and motherhood. The most popular image of a proper American woman in the late 1800s was one who was happily caring for her children in her home. These images and descriptions of smiling women with plump babies showed up in advertisements, in fiction, and in the writings of many elite physicians. Harvard physician Dr. Edward Clarke, in perhaps one of the most famous pamphlets on the issue, described the physical, emotional, and moral dangers to women who attempted to seek out higher education. He detailed case after case of young women's bodies and minds being wrecked by the physical trials (standing for long hours) and mental damage (all that reading!) of academic study. Each of his individual stories ended either as a cautionary tale—she was never able to have children—or as a lesson—after finally quitting her education, she was able to recuperate, marry, and have children.[2]

At the same time that Clarke and many others were trying to convince women of their biological imperative to stay at home and have children, scientists in America and Europe were publishing images of the peculiar, but universal, growing bodies involved in pregnancy. Evidence from embryology, the new science of human development *in utero*, was splashed all over the pages of popular health books, showed up in public museums and world's fairs, and could often be found in jars on the shelf of the local doctor's office. In the early nineteenth century many women would not have had much of an idea of what their developing fetuses looked like in their growing bellies, but their daughters and granddaughters could point to detailed drawings or wax models as evidence of what happens inside a pregnancy.

Upon embarking on this project, I assumed that the development of embryology and the intensification of mothering as a natural aspect of womanhood would craft miscarriage as a failure of womanhood, the death of a child, and perhaps even the fault of women. I rushed into the archives, thumbing through yellowed diaries and flaking letters from 150 years ago, certain I would find descriptions of grief, frustration, depression, or shame. Or maybe I would find nothing at all. Perhaps women of the nineteenth century kept quiet on the issue of miscarriage, feeling ashamed of their failures, or unable to discuss such a private, embarrassing topic.

What I discovered was unexpected and fascinating. I found women who were writing openly about their pregnancy losses and responding to the experience in a variety of ways. I found some women, as I expected, who were saddened by what they lost, frustrated by continued failure to have children, and disappointed in their bodies and reproductive fates. But I also found women relieved by their miscarriages, thankful for the event, and even happy afterward. At first this did not make sense. How could a woman who was attempting to fulfill her proper social (and national) role feel happy when she failed? As I sifted through personal papers of women who had been dead for over a hundred years, trying to imagine their lives, their emotions, and their circumstances, I began to understand how and why a woman would tell her mother she was thankful for a miscarriage; how and why a woman would inform her husband of the joy she felt after losing a pregnancy; how and why a young married woman could write in her diary that she was happy again after failing to become a mother. This chapter closely analyzes the writings of women—some who miscarried, others who gave birth to live infants—to provide insight into this bodily, familial, individual, and eventually medical event.

But these writings do not inform us only about reproducing in the past; they also inform us about current constructions and interpretations of reproduction. Scholars of twentieth-century pregnancy have often depicted the rise of fetal personification as being linked to visualization, culminating in ultrasounds and our current preoccupation with topics such as fetal pain and the lost babies (potential or present) involved in stem cell disposal. The links between the extent of fetal personification and modern technologies almost make it impossible to conceive that women living in an era before ultrasounds, IVF (in vitro fertilization), amniocentesis, and the ubiquitous fetal imagery around us could imagine an infant within their pregnant bellies. As I will examine in this chapter, women's writings refute this notion. Personal writings from the nineteenth century instead illuminate the fluidity of women's experiences with pregnancy at that time—the experience might include a child, a sense of ill health, or both, or even something in between. Investigating these writings allows us to analyze how depictions of pregnancy and miscarriage are involved in a complex web of fertility hopes, anxieties, limitations, and realities.

A Burden to Me: Having Children in the Nineteenth Century

Alice Kirk was no stranger to large families when she decided to marry childhood friend Ben Grierson in 1854. The oldest of thirteen, Kirk undoubtedly had a very good idea of what was involved in becoming a mother to many children. Her early married life, however, was perhaps not what she expected. Six years in, as the Civil War broke out, Ben Grierson was heavily in debt, and he had moved his family (Alice and two small boys) to live with his parents in Ohio. Enlisting in the army as a solution to the family's financial distress, Grierson quickly displayed his leadership skills and military acumen and rose in the ranks to major general by the end of the war. Following the war, Grierson was posted to various forts throughout the Western frontier, with his family always in tow. Alice Grierson followed her husband to Kansas, the Indian Territory, and then to the District of New Mexico, keeping house and caring for their ever-growing band of children.

In 1871, the family was stationed at Fort Sill, in Indian Territory, when their youngest child, a little girl named Mary Louisa, died

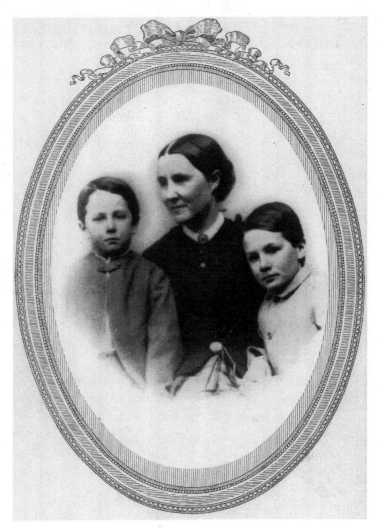

FIG. 1. Alice Kirk Grierson with two of her sons, most likely Charlie and Robert (ca. 1864). (Fort Davis National Historic Site)

at three months of age. This child was their seventh, and the grief from her death, along with health problems stemming from a difficult birth, drove Alice Grierson to her parents' home in Ohio to recuperate. Her husband did not seem happy with Alice's relocation, as he continually wrote to her asking when she would return to Fort Sill. Grierson replied, "There is no use in 'going it blind,' when we both have eyes to see, and commonsense to comprehend the facts of the case. Both of us will know one thing, which will inevitably occur, if the good Lord permits us to meet again, and are both well aware of the possible consequences which may follow. We are the temples of 'the living god,' and these temples must never again be desecrated by an incomplete act of worship (union)." In effect, Grierson was telling her husband that she was tired of getting pregnant, but she was not comfortable with one of the only methods of birth control available: withdrawal.

In a heartbreaking admission and peek into the reproductive realities that women in late nineteenth-century America experienced, Grierson then listed off her children and described how she felt at each pregnancy and birth:

> Charlie's existence I accepted as a matter of course, without either joy or sorrow. Kirkie's with regret, for so soon succeeding him. Robert came nearer being welcomed with joy, than any other. Edie was gladly welcomed so soon as I knew her sex. . . . Henry succeeded her too soon to give me as much rest as I would have liked . . . and told you before he was a year old, that I would rather die, than have another child, yet no sooner was he weaned, than Georgie came into life. . . . I firmly believe it injured me, as soon as I weaned him, and was again immediately pregnant, my nerves became so irritable to such a degree, that life has ever since, been nearer a burden to me.

After this litany, it is not surprising to read Grierson reporting that her nerves, after eleven years of such preparation, "have arrived at such a pitch of sensitiveness . . . [I] will need large, and long continued doses of rest, and quiet, to soothe them." Exhausted by a married life of never-ending reproduction, and perhaps remembering her mother in a similar situation, Grierson resorted to placing hundreds of miles between herself and her husband. This was the only way she could think of to put a stop to the pregnancies.[3]

Before reading these letters, I was well aware of the numbers and had heard the statistics showing families were large in nineteenth-century America (although also much smaller on average than they had been a century prior), but Grierson's letter makes the lived reality clear.[4] She was caught between a desire to space out her children but no effective means to accomplish this. By 1871, abortion was illegal in Ohio, birth control was becoming harder and harder to find (not to mention highly unreliable) and only a couple of years away from being outlawed, and even if Grierson had been amenable to these methods, living out in the Western frontier may have presented difficulties in accessing them.

Birthing children in nineteenth-century America was fraught with its own dangers, but women also faced increasing obstacles in their attempts to limit their childbearing. In 1873, the U.S. Congress passed the Comstock Act, which defined contraceptives and contraceptive information as obscene and thus illegal to send through the mail. Twenty-four states quickly passed their own laws placing prohibitions on the distribution, sale, and even use of such materials.[5] To be sure, contraception was not necessarily easy to obtain or highly effective before 1873. Couples could use any number of herbal remedies, such as tansy tea, to prevent conception or to "bring on the menses" of a woman who had stopped menstruating, with varying degrees of success. Some also used commercial devices, such as condoms made from animal skins or intestines and sponges. These devices, however, were expensive and difficult to find for many rural couples. Upon the development of the vulcanization of rubber in the 1840s, condoms, diaphragms, cervical caps, and douching syringes could now be constructed of rubber, driving down prices while increasing availability, ease of use, and durability. But this new market did not last long, as it was the promotion and sale of these new devices—in newspapers, mail-order catalogs, and in dry-goods stores—that motivated many legislators to seek the illegalization of contraception.[6]

Abortion was also under threat in the second half of the nineteenth century. Although many states had some sort of abortion law on the books in the first half of the century, most of those followed British common law and stipulated the procedure as illegal only after quickening (the first movements of the fetus felt by the mother, typically at around four months). In the 1860s, however, regular physicians viewed the illegalization of abortion at any time during pregnancy as a good way to push midwives out of the market, thus increasing their patient base and raising their professional status. Because of a large-scale effort by a small group of elite physicians led by Boston doctor Horatio Storer, by 1880 most states had passed laws outlawing abortion from the time of conception.[7]

Between 1860 and 1900, American women faced growing restrictions on their control over fertility, and yet they also found ways to limit the size of their families, as the fertility rate dropped from 5.42 children per family in 1850 to 3.56 in 1900.[8] Families accomplished this by physical separation, as was the case with the Griersons, by using common household products as birth control (such as vinegar douches), by illegal abortions, and by delaying marriage. Historians, too, often neglect the paradox of these two trends: family size decreased at the same time as obstacles to legal, safe, and effective methods for fertility control increased. Instead, we need to ponder what those simultaneous trends can tell us about the desire, perhaps even desperation, of women to stop having children.

It is within this context of the difficulty, but deep desire, of many nineteenth-century women to limit their fertility that we can better understand miscarriage reactions. Subsequently, the analysis of women's writings about miscarriage complicates common conceptions of nineteenth-century femininity. There is a rich literature in gender history exposing the intensifying link between motherhood and womanhood toward the end of the century—this was partially a response to women's growing presence in higher education, the workforce, and the public sphere more generally.[9] Following this claim (which I am not disputing), it would be reasonable to assume that doctors and women would interpret miscarriage as a failure of motherhood and thus a failure of femininity, as they often did with infertility.[10]

Although historians have perhaps anachronistically assumed motherhood to automatically include pregnancy, this investigation into miscarriage calls into question that very link. Despite established connections between womanhood and motherhood in the late nineteenth century, neither women's reactions to miscarriage nor medical discussions of pregnancy loss employed a language of failure or blame. Such an omission encourages us to reconsider the category and meaning of motherhood, especially in its relationship to pregnancy. A failed pregnancy was not necessarily viewed as failed womanhood, even if producing children was considered the primary role for women.

As women like Alice Grierson found themselves living in a new world that limited their control over pregnancy or child spacing, this highly restrictive reproductive world also created a space of freedom when it came to miscarriage. In what seems to be a contradiction, while doctors, politicians, and popular writers informed women that their sole duty in life was to have children, and their lives should be shaped around that undertaking, when that enterprise failed in the form of miscarriage, no one blamed the woman, least of all herself. As I will show later, doctors instead looked to uncontrollable conditions, common aspects of life, or neglected to consider causation at all. In turn, women responded to their miscarriages, not in accordance with some larger social role or message, but within the context of their own personal desires and family plans. This chapter, through the analysis of four individual women, will illustrate both the various factors involved in the interpretation of miscarriage, and also the relative freedom American women felt at choosing how to respond to the event. This shaping of miscarriage into a common, often welcomed, but mostly benign occurrence also influenced the understanding of pregnancy. If a woman was relieved that she had a miscarriage, she was perhaps less likely to imagine a baby within her body. While nineteenth-century women were not as interested in determining the personhood status of the objects contained within pregnancy as we might be today, we can still glean some understanding of what kinds of bodies—in terms of both maternal and fetal—existed in pregnancy.

Another Sitka Baby

Emily McCorkle came from an old, distinguished Pennsylvania family; she was born on land that had been purchased from William Penn himself. As was proper for her station, she attended Miss Dicken's School for Girls in Harrisburg, surely thought to be excellent training for her future as a wife and mother. In 1872, McCorkle embarked on that future when she married Jenkins FitzGerald, an army surgeon. The FitzGeralds were soon stationed at West Point, and a year later the couple welcomed their first child, Elizabeth, whom the family called Bess. Shortly after, her husband received new orders sending them to Sitka, Alaska, and Emily FitzGerald began to pack up their house. In 1874, a three-months-pregnant FitzGerald boarded a ship in New York with her toddler and her husband, setting sail for what was truly the edge of the American frontier. The family sailed to Panama, trekked for three hours across land, and boarded another ship bound for San Francisco. FitzGerald reported to her mother, back in Pennsylvania, almost daily of their journey, describing her seasickness, and her growing worry that they would not reach their new home before she gave birth. While stopped in Portland, Oregon, FitzGerald wrote, "I hope I have not counted wrong about the time to be sick. As it is, I have just about time to get to Sitka and fixed up."[11] She did make it to Sitka, having time to direct workers on repainting the family rooms, sew clothes for the coming baby, and attempt to wrangle her "scamp" of a daughter before giving birth to Herbert in late October.[12]

The following year, FitzGerald was again pregnant. The letters to her mother that fall do not depict a comfortable life. On November 10, 1875, she reported, "Such a horrid month as we have had! I have been worried about Bess's eyes, I have been sick myself, and a hundred disagreeable things have happened." In that same letter, FitzGerald described the labor of a fellow army wife: "She has a boy, a great, big fellow . . . poor child, her troubles are just beginning." Two weeks later, FitzGerald wrote of her own troubles: "I have not been feeling well for a month. I know I look badly and

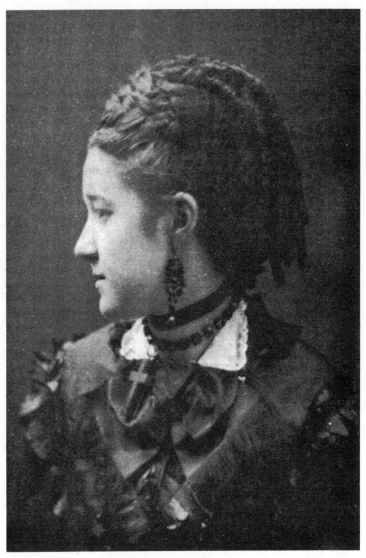

FIG. 2. Emily McCorkle FitzGerald (undated).

I know Doctor has been a little concerned, for he has put me on cod liver oil, and iron and quinine, and all those lovely things. I did not think I would tell you until I saw you, but I will now. I had a miscarriage about five or six weeks ago, but I lost a great deal of blood and all my strength . . . I have not gotten over it yet." Like

Mary Longfellow, FitzGerald suffered in the wake of her miscarriage, which was a concern to her husband, and perhaps she knew that such a tale would worry her mother.[13]

While FitzGerald made no direct remarks in her previous letters about keeping her family small, or desiring more space between her children (the first two being only a year apart), her feelings about the miscarriage were very clear in the letter: "I am thankful now that I did have it, as another Sitka baby would have been my fate." FitzGerald was not pleased at the prospect of raising another child in the harsh environment of her home. Her letters were full of problems she had with the "girl" hired to help with the children, her difficulties in getting materials for clothing for her growing children, conflicts with native populations, and her constant fatigue over maintaining a house and a life in such a cold, unforgiving region. "I guess the climate has a good deal to do with it," she wrote her mother concerning her lingering illness.[14]

While not perhaps explicitly stating her desires to limit her fertility, FitzGerald did make mention of her attempts at some measure of control. She informed her mother that while she may no longer be pregnant now, her sister Sallie "need not trouble herself to have any. I can supply the family. I don't believe there is any safe day in the month for me. Indeed, I know there isn't—15th—16th—17th—or any other." This line reveals that while she may not have taken purposeful measures to prevent pregnancy, FitzGerald was keeping track of when she had sex and if she got pregnant—a practice most commonly used when trying to avoid pregnancy.[15] FitzGerald apparently had not been the only woman in Sitka who was attempting to control her family size, or who was at least concerned over her seeming fecundity as she continued, "Mrs. Campbell, Mrs. Field, and I have meetings of horror over the subject, as we have all gone through so much together here and we all seem to be awfully prolific."[16]

While Emily FitzGerald may not have clearly stated that her relief over her miscarriage was a direct result of the growing restrictions placed on women's attempts to control fertility, we cannot discount that she was trying to track her pregnancy and was not very happy about her fruitful body. Both her family situation—already having two young children, which appeared to be exhausting for her—and her physical environment—an Alaskan island, over 800 miles from the nearest American town—created a situation in which miscarriage was perhaps the only recourse from further suffering and struggle. FitzGerald was not a wealthy woman, with servants to care for her house and nannies for her children. She was trying to make a life and a family in a harsh environment, with limited social support, and meager financial resources.

FitzGerald's letters introduce the idea that individual American women understood their miscarriages in very situationally specific ways. Economics, environment, family structure, social support, personal desires, and health all played important roles in women's determinations of how to respond to, or describe, a miscarriage. The individual women in this book reveal a wide variety of experiences and responses, but as a group they exhibit a broader ambivalence to the event.

I Am Happy Again

In 1862, Annie Youmans sat down to write, "My sister Charlotte and I have commenced to write a journal today I am fourteen years old. Charlotte is sixteen. Mary Ellenor is past nineteen, Laura is eight my dear little brother is twenty three months old and Ma and Pa between forty three and four years old. That is as large as our family is. It has been raining all day."[17] For the next nineteen years, Youmans continued this writing, often detailing activities of her family and the weather. Ten years in, Youmans's writings revolved around multiple young men, including even a description of a short-lived engagement to Edward De l'Ouest. By the spring of 1873, however, one particular man appeared more often than the others, and on April 27 she wrote, "Well I am not engaged just yet, but suppose I am as good as it, for Mr Van Ness asked me to marry him to night. I dont mean he wanted me to marry him to night but I mean that it was to night he asked me, I wouldn't give him any decided answer, but I suppose I shall have to say Yes sometime I told him he would have to become a Christian before I would consent." One of You-mans's hesitations came from the fact that Mr. Van Ness was a widower with a young son, a situation that caused her to write, "the idea of . . . being a step mother, how comical!"[18]

Youmans seemed to take pleasure in her power over her possi-ble intended, writing a month later, "I wont be married till a year from June at least . . . I shall have a good time making Mr Van Ness wait so long contentedly for he is beginning to beg for next winter already, but I tell him if he isn't a mind to wait he can go and marry somebody else, and he is docile immediately." While Youmans spent most of the summer meeting her intended's vari-ous family members and slowly letting her own sisters and parents in on the secret, Theodore Van Ness was preoccupied with finan-cial matters. In September 1873, Youmans described his troubles: "my journal, it is when I feel blue and need consolation that I come to you, that is partly the case now although it is not on my own account, but for Theodore, this Wall St smash up has affected him as he had almost every thing he had invested in stocks, so of course lost with the rest." Van Ness had waited to tell her, she reported, "for fear it would alter my love for him, the idea! he must have thought I only cared for his money, well perhaps I gave him the impression, I know now that I do love him and will try to be a comfort and help to him instead of a useless clog of a wife, poor fellow I feel so sorry for him."[19]

Annie Youmans and Theodore Van Ness were married on October 8, 1873. For the first few years, Van Ness wrote often of the economizing measures they were taking, including having to move from New York City to Yonkers, New York, as was more fitting to their new financial situation. One of the habits Van Ness adopted was to close out her diary for the year with a note detailing the amount of money she spent that year. In 1872, the total was $142.32, and in 1873, the year of her wedding, the amount was $363.26. The first full year of her marriage, Van Ness spent only $68.48. This reduction in her wealth might explain why, in January 1875, when she suspected she was pregnant, Van Ness reported that the condi-tion made her "very cross and irritable and I think I have very good reason to feel ill humored." The following month, she reported, "I dont know that I am in much better humor than when I last wrote as the cause of it, still exists."[20]

Two weeks later, Van Ness's mood was much altered: "Quite a change has come over the spirit of my dream since last I wrote, and I am happy again, a week ago last night I was taken sick at the supper table, I went to my room and retired early, to make a long story short I will say, that the next day Ma told me she had seen her first grand child." Van Ness quickly amended the report: "I just happened to think that any body might imagine from reading this that I had a baby, but I haven't! it was only what they call a miss—."[21]

Van Ness allows us another view into miscarrying in the nineteenth century in how she describes the products of her pregnancy loss. Contemporary debates inform us that women are more likely to understand their pregnancies as inclusive of a child if they can see the childlike figure within their bodies. Additionally, a woman should mourn a miscarriage or abortion if what she delivers resembles a child. Van Ness described what she delivered not only as her mother's first grandchild, but also added: "it wasn't any larger than a jointed doll." Comparing the miscarriage products to a doll indicates that Van Ness saw a material body that contained humanistic parts and form, but she still described herself as feeling "pretty smart" after the event. Like FitzGerald, Van Ness viewed her miscarriage as a positive experience. As a young wife living in Yonkers in the wake of the economic depression, Van Ness may not have been ready for the cost and responsibility of a child. Instead, her situation caused her to see the miscarriage as welcomed and a cause for relief.

The Imaginary Number 10

It was not only the struggle of life in the wilds of the Alaskan frontier, or the economic downturn that led American women to find relief in miscarriage; sometimes the reasons were more commonplace. Mary Bushnell, daughter of influential minister and theologian Horace Bushnell, married Frank Cheney in 1863.

Cheney, along with two brothers, had begun experimenting with silk production in the 1830s, and by 1860 he had built a business that boasted 600 workers and annual production over $500,000.[22] Frank and Mary settled down in Hartford, Connecticut, where Mary soon got to work building a family while Frank traveled the country promoting silk. Having given birth to their first child, Emily, only eleven months after their wedding, Mary embarked on the next twenty years in a state of near constant reproduction.

In June 1879, Mary Cheney wrote a letter to her husband, Frank, revealing her latest pregnancy. By then, the Cheneys had been married for sixteen years and had nine children. Mary described this pregnancy to her husband: "I was not mistaken about myself when you went away. But it is all right. I am feeling perfectly well and everyone says I look so. I really believe this is getting to be my normal condition."[23] Mary joked about a condition that was common for many nineteenth-century women: twenty or thirty years of constant pregnancy, birthing, and nursing.

The following month, she updated her husband about her condition, describing the loss of the pregnancy by beginning the letter, "O Bliss, O Rapture unforeseen!" She explained: "the imaginary Number 10, whom I had already begun to love, is not a real entity as yet, and I hope will not be for a long time to come."[24] To further explain the situation, Cheney added, "I don't know that we are called on to mourn the loss of a child, but you will perhaps wonder at me that I found it at first so hard to part with my trial—for trial it had been but one in which much sweetness had been hidden."[25] I struggled with this entry at first: could I accurately term this a miscarriage, or was it a case of delayed menstruation? Then I realized that distinction may not have been a meaningful one to Cheney, or to many women in nineteenth-century America.[26] The ambiguity of early pregnancy (as I will detail in the next chapter), as well as the ambiguity of available language for early pregnancy, means we can only read Cheney's statement as: there was a perceived pregnancy, but it slipped away. Without modern urine tests and ultrasounds, nineteenth-century women relied on changeable

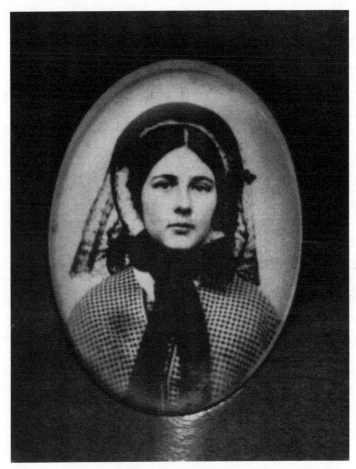

FIG. 3. Mary Cheney (ca. early 1860s). (Cheney Family Papers, Sophia Smith Collection, Smith College, Northampton, Mass.)

and indeterminate symptoms to decide if they were pregnant. Women benefitted from this ambiguity between early pregnancy and delayed menstruation, not only because they may not have been able to tell the difference, but also because they may not have desired the pregnancy.[27] Cheney's personal situation—a mother of nine with the youngest only nine months old—created a context that produced a lost pregnancy that could at once be a thing to mourn and a thing to celebrate.

These positive reactions to miscarriage remind us that, while in today's world miscarriage may be primarily regarded as an event of sadness, loss, and failure, that notion is shaped by the ability of most women to have a measure of control over their fertility. I do not mean to argue that every woman today feels sadness or loss in the wake of a miscarriage. Rather, I mean that the predominant narrative for miscarriage (appearing everywhere from popular magazines to medical literature and parenting guides) includes these sentiments, although this narrative (like many mainstream stories we tell about "women") refers primarily to middle- and upper-class white women. In late nineteenth-century America, women had much less control over when and how many pregnancies they had, and so miscarriage was more likely to be a relief, very welcomed, or a reason to celebrate. Emily FitzGerald had no desire to bring another child into the harsh and unforgiving environment of the Alaskan frontier; Annie Van Ness was grappling with a troublesome stepson and may not have seen a way to afford a new infant; even Mary Cheney, living a comfortable upper-class life in Connecticut, had her hands quite full with her large family and saw little pleasure in another pregnancy. It is within this context that we can better understand why, even in the face of intensifying pressure to become mothers, nineteenth-century women could openly discuss the relief of a miscarriage.

I Am Sincerely Sorry for It

To be sure, not all women experiencing miscarriage in the nineteenth century were overjoyed at the event. The stories of Emily FitzGerald, Annie Van Ness, and Mary Cheney illustrate how the increasing restrictions on reproductive life in late nineteenth-century America shaped women's interpretations of their pregnancies and their miscarriages. But this was not the only response; in order to fully understand miscarriage in the nineteenth century, I will turn to another example, that of Ella Gertrude Clanton Thomas, a woman who miscarried early in her reproductive life, and who expressed no joy, but may have longed for a miscarriage by the end of her childbearing years. Thomas reveals just how situationally constructed miscarriage interpretations could be; even in the same woman, personal situations, family economics, or social standing could change and in turn alter how a woman felt about her fertile body and what was developing inside.

The daughter of one of the wealthiest planters in Georgia, Gertrude Clanton was accustomed to the genteel life in the antebellum South. In 1849 at the age of fourteen, Clanton left home to attend the Wesleyan Female College in Macon, Georgia, joining a small minority of elite Southern women entering higher education. In her three years there, Clanton strengthened her Methodist beliefs and made several lifelong friends, including Julia Thomas. Soon after her graduation from Wesleyan, Gertrude began receiving the attentions of Thomas's brother, Jefferson, seeing in him everything she could wish for in a spouse: wealth, social standing, and respectability. Although Jefferson Thomas brought his own financial stability to the marriage, when the couple wed in 1852, Clanton's father gifted them with a house, plantation, and slaves worth almost $30,000.[28]

Gertrude Thomas quickly became pregnant, giving birth to their son, Turner, within the first year, and then giving birth every two to three years for the next twenty years. When little Turner was eighteen months old, Thomas determined she was pregnant again, writing in her journal: "I am again destined to be a mother." Reflecting on this new addition, Thomas admitted that because her pregnancy was causing her constant headaches and a sick stomach, she could not yet "view the idea with a great deal of interest or pleasure."[29] A few months later, Thomas's writings reveal a much-improved state of health and subsequently more excitement for the coming child. Tragically, her second son, Joseph, died only three weeks after his birth. Seven months later, Thomas was again pregnant: "Again, I have prospects of becoming a mother and the idea . . . causes pleasurable emotions." A month later, however, Thomas miscarried, discussing the event in her journal primarily in terms of her physical health: "I have been sick two weeks and feel as tho I had been ill two months."[30]

Her next pregnancy, coming five months later, Thomas described with joy: "I am very happy in the prospect . . . and hope that I may do my duty as a mother to the immortal soul entrusted to my care."[31] Over the next six years, Thomas gave birth three more times, losing one daughter after only seven months. While she continued to experience "sick stomach" and headaches with all her pregnancies, Thomas welcomed each child and mourned greatly when little Anna Lou died so young. By 1863, however, the family's income and social circumstances had begun to take a turn for the worse. When the Civil War first broke out, Gertrude Thomas, like many elite women in the South, championed the Confederate cause and gloried in her husband's military service. By 1864, however, she found the shortages, inflation, and social instability less exciting and taking a toll on her physical and mental health. When she discovered she was pregnant in December 1862, Thomas described her feelings as: "I cannot say blessed with the prospect of again becoming a mother." By February 1865, while waiting for the expected approach of the Union army, Thomas described her latest pregnancy as decidedly unwelcomed: "unfortunately I have a prospect of again adding to the little members of my household—of again becoming a mother . . . I am sincerely sorry for it."[32]

Gertrude Thomas gave birth to ten children over the course of twenty-two years, and more than once she remarked in her journal of her wish to space out those children a bit more. Upon determining she was pregnant for the third time, Thomas wrote that she would "not object to long intervals" between pregnancies.[33] While Georgia would not enact its stringent antiabortion law until 1876, and the Comstock Law was still years away, Thomas lived in a social world where a woman of her station should not have considered actively preventing pregnancy. This lack of control along with the upheaval brought on by the Civil War may have contributed to Thomas's observation that her later pregnancies were less and less "pleasurable" or "blessed." Although Thomas did not express clear joy or relief in her early miscarriage, her writings do reveal how each of a woman's pregnancies could be differently construed, reminding us of how often today, despite the rhetoric of the antiabortion movement drawing clear lines between women who are mothers and women who abort pregnancies, in reality pregnancy loss or termination and motherhood often coexist for the same woman.

What or Who

Analyzing these personal writings that describe pregnancy and miscarriage reveal not only the variety of reactions to miscarriage, but also the diversity in how women interpreted their pregnant bodies. These letters and diaries can expose how particular women thought about pregnancy, motherhood, their role in their family and their community, and how all of these aspects shaped their understanding of the changes taking place in their bodies. These writings also raise new questions about our modern understandings of pregnancy, fetus, and child. While nineteenth-century American women may not have understood their pregnancies in terms of an infant or fetus within the womb as women might today, these descriptions nevertheless reveal new links among fertility control, social definitions of motherhood, and the embodied experiences of pregnancy and miscarriage.

Lucy McKim Garrison was three months pregnant and had already named her child Katherine. Garrison wrote a thank-you note to her in-laws using the voice of her unborn daughter. "Katherine" assured her grandparents that she welcomed the Christmas present of a pair of socks, even though she could not say "that she was suffering from cold feet just at that time." Katherine also sent "a Happy New Year to her kind Grandparents" and expressed her plan to knit them something some future Christmas—a plan that would have to wait because "her fingers [were] not yet her own to do [with] as she please[d]."[34]

This charming note may strike readers as unsurprising in an early twenty-first-century world that uses fetal images in advertising, consults pregnancy websites detailing "baby's" weekly development, and faces an abortion debate that often highlights the similarities between a three-month fetus and a full-term infant. But Garrison wrote this letter in 1866. In a time long before women could "see" their pregnancies through ultrasounds, or even "know" that they were pregnant with the help of a urine test, Lucy Garrison imagined her daughter existing in her body, complete with warm feet and uncontrollable fingers. Ending the letter with her own report that "the child has hardly left me room for a word, what a talker at so early an age!" Garrison interpreted her pregnant body as one that included another person with body parts and actions. Unfortunately, perhaps, for Garrison, "Katherine" became Lloyd upon his birth, although Katherine did come along six years later.[35] Garrison presents an endearing example of what we would now term the "personification" of pregnancy (a word that Garrison and most intellectuals in the nineteenth century would never have considered), but this is just one instance. As with their interpretations of miscarriage, nineteenth-century women showed a wide range of interpretations of pregnancy, each constructed according to personal, social, and cultural circumstances.

For some women, the pregnant body was an ill body. Gertrude Thomas commonly described her pregnancies in the 1850s in terms of "sickness," "debility," and "suffering."[36] Ellen Wright Garrison reported to her sister in 1879 about missing a family wedding: "I was too deadly sick to go! Six weeks along & can't swallow a morsel but gruel & the like! . . . I can't go near the table, or even sit straight in a chair, but have to lie down nearly all the time!"[37] Many women recorded their pregnancy experiences in terms of sickness or as a condition that sapped their energy or made them feel unwell.[38]

But for some, illness was only the beginning of what was developing within their pregnant bodies. Many nineteenth-century American women admitted that something existed in their expanding bodies, and that thing frequently moved. Four months into her pregnancy, Elizabeth Cabot recorded in 1865 that she could "feel motion for the first time—almost imperceptible."[39] While today descriptions of quickening are typically framed around the kicks of an imagined baby, in the nineteenth century this movement was often chronicled in more abstract, depersonalized terms. Such descriptions may have been the result of how a woman felt about a particular pregnancy. Alice Kirk Grierson wrote to her husband during her sixth pregnancy, "I am very sure that since my arrival here, I have *felt* positive indications that we may make our calculations for the arrival of a young stranger by midsummer."[40] Years later, Grierson would remark that she dreaded each pregnancy, especially beginning with this one, her sixth.[41] Writing of quickening as "positive indications" rather than motions of a sentient being may have been Grierson's way of facing a less-than-desired pregnancy.

While scholars have considered historical references to quickening primarily in discussions of pregnancy determination or the criminalization of abortion, descriptions of this phenomenon in personal writings also provide an important window into women's understanding of what was happening inside of their bodies. In 1838, Mary Walker described the motion as "the leaping." This word choice could be a reflection of her spiritual inclinations (in the Bible when Elizabeth was pregnant with John the Baptist, the child "leaped" in her womb), but it also could indicate that she considered the motion an action by a body that could move like a child. Walker also wrote that she was "happy in anticipating" her future child, which perhaps was a reason she did not use the more generic, depersonalized term "motion."[42]

Blanche Butler Ames was pregnant at least six times between 1871 and 1882, and from the first pregnancy she paid special attention to how her body felt and how it might appear to others. Ames's husband, Adelbert (Del), lived apart from the family while he served as a U.S. senator and then governor of Mississippi, resulting in a large collection of letters between the couple. In May 1871, while six months pregnant, Blanche Ames described the behavior of the creature within her after she had spent the day gardening: "it was quite unruly, and would not hesitate to kick its parents, if such a thing were possible."[43] Her choice of "kicking" brings to mind the modern usage of the word and its connection to images of fetal feet found on ultrasounds, but Ames's qualification allows us to see our modern, implied meaning of "kick"—as a purposeful action by a sentient being. For Ames, however, what was inside her was not necessarily a person, as she could not conceive of "it"

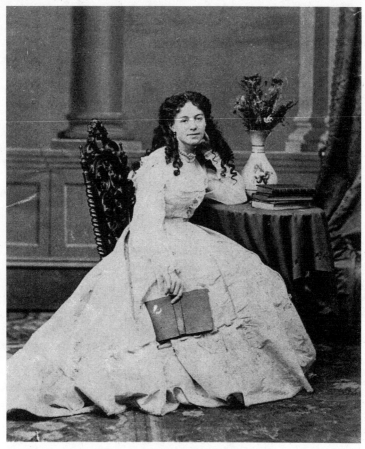

FIG. 4. Blanche Butler Ames (1865). (Ames Family Papers, Sophia Smith Collection, Smith College, Northampton, Mass.)

kicking others. Thus, while women may have conceptualized the being housed in pregnancy as something that moved and grew, they did not necessarily consider it a distinct body or person.

When she was pregnant with her third child in 1874, Ames took to weighing herself as a way to keep track of her bodily changes. She reported to Del: "I was weighed again today, and would you believe it, Del, I have gained seven pounds since I came down here? Of course, all of the flesh is not upon <u>my</u> bones. Still no doubt I have my fair share."[44] Ames recognized that there could be bones of another body inside of her, but her words indicate more of a grey area than we tend to consider in modern conceptions of pregnancy. The movement and bones inside of her uterus perhaps did not comprise a body, and yet not quite *not* a body. Like many of the women considered here, Ames instead described a more ambiguous concept of her pregnancy. There was something inside of her uterus, but she felt little compulsion to decide whether it was a body or a person. The nineteenth century was instead an era in which women could understand the development within their pregnant bodies on their own terms, without reference to scientific revelations or medical conceptions.

Some women, meanwhile, were quite eager to depict their pregnant bodies as housing children. Lucy McKim Garrison wrote to her childhood friend-cum-sister-in-law, Ellen Wright Garrison, in 1874 of the coming of her fourth child. She wrote of her children, two sons and two daughters: "Perhaps you hadn't heard of two girls. Well, there are two; one you have seen and the other you shall see when you come to pay us a visit next June."[45] Two months into her pregnancy, Garrison was already writing about the existence—not just the future—of a daughter. This was the same woman who wrote a thank-you note in the voice of her unborn child.[46] Even probably before feeling movement inside, Garrison imagined a female infant residing within her body.

Other women were quite willing to convey their pregnancies as inclusive of a person. In 1880, Ellen Wright Garrison described her pregnancy to her sister, Eliza Wright Osborne: "It is good fun, getting ready for Eleanor, & people send me lovely things!"[47] Garrison, who had already named her future child, wrote in a way to indicate she already thought of her fetus as a person, two months before its birth. Rather than a pregnancy that entailed a creature within her womb, Garrison described a daughter.

Lucy Garrison's habit of discussing her pregnancies in terms of children did not become a family custom. Garrison's daughter, Katherine, instead referred to her unborn child as a genderless object. In an 1898 letter to her cousin, Katherine Garrison Norton described her pregnancy as "the presence of a little Norton which (since it won't be a 'who' until December) makes any more traveling than is absolutely necessary rather risky."[48] Norton did not imagine a son or daughter in her womb, but she indicated that birth would transform the unborn into a humanized baby.

These findings illuminate the complexity of fetal personification, as well as the fluidity in imagining what kind of body might be involved in pregnancy. Some described a particular person inside of their wombs, whereas others clearly resisted doing so. For some women, the habit of describing pregnancy in abstract and depersonalized terms may have been connected to a history of miscarriage and infant death, but this was not the case for Katherine Norton, who was pregnant for the first time when she wrote her cousin. In an era that historians often describe as restrictive, both in terms of reproductive control and women's roles, this research reveals the freedom nineteenth-century women displayed in terms of their individual interpretations of pregnancy.

By the close of the nineteenth century, American women encountered multiple opportunities to "see" the tiny beings contained in pregnancy, and yet women like Katherine Norton still did not think of their pregnant bodies as containing a person, calling into question the historical connections between fetal visualization and fetal personification. Scholars have argued that the "cult of fetal personhood" emerged in the past fifty years, partially because of new visualization technologies.[49] The ability to see the human fetus in a new light—spurred on by Lennart Nilsson's classic series of photographs of fetal development printed in *Life* magazine in 1965, and sustained by the availability of ultrasound images—has resulted in a new understanding of human development. Scholars contend that these technological transformations also altered the relationship between a pregnant woman and her fetus, and also between the fetus and the public.[50]

The personal writings included here demonstrate that the connection between visualizing the fetus and personifying it was neither a simple nor inevitable one.[51] By the 1870s, when embryology was entering the public consciousness through museum and fair displays as well as popular health literature, women continued to describe their pregnancies in a wide variety of ways—some indicating a person inside, and some steering clear of such constructions. Markedly different from our current obsession with "the baby" inside the bump, nineteenth-century women's understanding of what was inside their bodies was more fluid. For some women, it was a person in the making, and for others it was a more nebulous object, or an object that became a person only at birth.

Blanche Ames presents us with one reason why the popularization of embryology did not automatically lead women to imagine a developing baby within their pregnant bodies. In 1871, she was five months pregnant and took a walk with her father, perhaps looking for some relief from feeling "cumbersome" during her first pregnancy. As they came upon a pond, Ames later reported in a letter to her husband, "I remarked upon the funny look of the tadpoles, with their great heads and little tails. To my astonishment Father said 'Why, don't you know you began in just that way?'" Ames admitted to being skeptical, "Do you suppose, Del, human beings, while being formed, ever wriggle around like tadpoles? Alas, for human vanity, if such is the case!"[52] Ames, perhaps like many women, was not comfortable with the thought that what was growing inside her body was akin to a tadpole. Even though nineteenth-century scientists began showing proof to the public of the fetal bodies created by and contained throughout pregnancy, these bodies did not always look like human infants. In his 1875 *Ladies' Medical Guide*, Philadelphia physician and professor Seth Pancoast detailed fetal development, including an illustration of the embryo at thirty days that could easily be mistaken for a fish or a tadpole, along with the remark, "On the thirtieth day the embryo is about the size of a horse-fly, and looks something like a worm that is bent."[53] While the new science of embryology sought to show women that pregnant bodies did in fact contain developing human bodies, many women undoubtedly viewed these bodies as animalistic or eerily similar to insects, prompting little change in their behavior.

These personal writings unveil the complexity of nineteenth-century pregnancy. While historians have examined the ambiguity of pregnancy experiences in the early modern era and the eighteenth century, too often they have assumed that this ambiguity disappeared with the growth of embryology.[54] Once doctors and the public could *see* what the developing human looked like, then surely they viewed pregnancy with more precision and began to conceive of the condition as inclusive of a small person. Nineteenth-century writings by women such as Lucy Garrison, Blanche Ames, and Katherine Norton complicate historians' assumptions by demonstrating instead a consistency of ambiguity about pregnancy.

Conclusion

In nineteenth-century America, miscarriage stood as an occasion for celebration, a tragedy to mourn, a normal part of female reproduction, and an abnormal occurrence to be fixed by male physicians. Unraveling the connections among these contradictory categories reveals new insight into what it meant to be a woman in this world. But closer analysis also uncovers the social, cultural, economic, and medical forces that shape the phenomenon of miscarriage, in the nineteenth century and today. By focusing in on the personal stories of women such as Annie Van Ness, we can get a snapshot of how women juggled their personal anxieties, family desires, and everyday battles. Van Ness's experience also provides insight into how entwined women's reproductive realities were with economic considerations, social concerns, and cultural constructions of family and health.

In the following four chapters, I will delve deeper into the abilities of nineteenth-century American women to determine their reproductive destinies, their responses to miscarriage, and their understandings of how medicine could help or hurt them. At the same time, I will detail the emergence of professional medical interest in miscarriage. Why did regular physicians begin to pay attention to what previously had been understood as common and natural? What were physicians hoping to gain by convincing women that miscarriage was a medical problem to fix? As I trace miscarriage over the course of the nineteenth century, I will argue that growing medical interest in miscarriage was driven by doctors' interests in professional status and scientific research, enabled by national social and racial changes, and continually shaped by miscarrying women. Only by closely examining the words of individual women upon detecting the signs of a miscarriage, in the midst of a miscarriage, or in the wake of a miscarriage can we ascertain the power of lay women to shape a reproductive world that was increasingly becoming defined by scientific medicine.

2

Enveloped in Mystery

Pregnancy and Miscarriage in the Late Eighteenth and Early Nineteenth Centuries

In 1777, Abigail Adams's life was in turmoil, to put it lightly. Her young country was at war, and her husband, John, was in Baltimore with Congress, leaving Abigail at home in Massachusetts with their four children—a situation Abigail was quite used to by then. In March of that year, Congress moved to Philadelphia, a city in the direct path of the advancing British army. While caring for her children, the family farm, and worrying over the health and life of her husband, Abigail Adams also discovered she was pregnant for the sixth time (two-year-old "Suky" had died in 1770). After feeling ill for most of the pregnancy, struggling with insomnia and an early heat wave, Adams wrote to her husband on July 9 that on the previous evening she had been "taken with a shaking fit" and was "very apprehensive that a life was lost." Writing, "I have no reason to day to think otherwise," she relayed her belief that the pregnancy would not be successful.[1] Experienced with pregnancy, Adams read the internal signs of her body to determine that her pregnancy was over, and another child was not forthcoming. However, Adams still called a doctor to corroborate her suspicions. As she reported to her husband: "the Dr. encourages me to Hope that my apprehensions are groundless respecting what I wrote you yesterday." While perhaps viewing the physician as some sort of expert, at least enough of one to seek out in the case of a shaking fit, Adams did not trust in his diagnosis of her pregnancy, writing: "I cannot say I have had any reason to alter my mind."[2]

Adams relied on the signs she received from her body to suspect that her pregnancy would be lost, but her physician, a gentleman seeking to gain legitimacy as a male authority, disregarded this personal, female bodily expertise. While influenced perhaps by her class or the professional status of her husband (a graduate of Harvard, a lawyer, and a member of Congress in this new nation) to seek out a doctor in the case of a miscarriage, Adams felt no need to trust in his expertise over her own corporeal experience. The doctor, relying on external signs he could read on her body, did not know, after all, what it felt like to be pregnant, and what it felt like for that pregnancy to come to an end. As she disclosed five days later, "my apprehensions with regard to it were well founded ... [and] I was perfectly sensible of its disease as I even before was of its existence."[3] In the end, the medical advice proved ineffectual and a misdiagnosis. Adams herself knew what was happening with her body, but she was forced to wait until it could be exposed to others before her doctor would agree.

Dating back to at least the eighteenth century, American woman and physicians conferred over cases of miscarriage, each bringing to the encounter their individual interpretations of the event, personal or professional expertise, and socially influenced interests. By the end of the nineteenth century, these interactions would result in the coproduction of embryological knowledge and changes in medical treatment, but in 1777 these exchanges more often resulted in conflict over bodily knowledge. Abigail Adams relied on the sensations she felt, or ceased to feel, deep within her body to determine both the presence and the end of her pregnancy. Her doctor, in turn, having no means to access the internal workings of her body, was instead forced to rely on external signs. This differential knowledge created interactions that could result in the appearance of medical incompetence and the triumph of female bodily expertise. While early nineteenth-century scientific and philosophical shifts in understandings of pregnancy would end up transforming miscarriage from a natural fix into a medical puzzle, giving physicians a glimmer of authority over miscarriage as part of their expanding medical oversight of reproduction in reality doctors repeatedly left patients unconvinced of their expertise.[4]

Useless Beings: Conceptions of Pregnancy under Preformation

In 1749, Johann Storch, a physician living and practicing in the German town of Eisenach, published an eight-volume set on women's health, based on his forty years of experience as a practitioner. He titled the fourth volume *Diseases of Women Wherein Primarily Such Mishaps as Concerns Lumps, Womb Growths or Fake Fruits are Discussed Theoretically and Practically*.[5] As suggested by the long, but informative title, this volume centered on the vast array of "objects" a doctor might find within (or more likely would find expelled by) the female womb, all of which were decidedly not children. He recounted case after case in which a female patient believed herself pregnant, only to deliver "bubbly lots," "untoward matter," "fleshy morsels," and "useless beings."[6] Another German physician, Wilhelm Gottfried von Ploucquet, affirmed in 1788, "not everything that comes from the birth parts of a woman is a human being."[7]

The idea that the human uterus could house entities within it that bore little relation to a human infant was by no means a new idea by the eighteenth century, nor was it restricted to German physicians. Many Western medical thinkers and women discussed the idea of false conception or the growth of "moles."[8] Just because a woman ceased to menstruate, felt tenderness in her breasts, and noticed her abdomen expanding, she could not be assured that she was truly pregnant. These signs instead could signal the growth of a mole or some other useless being. Prior to the middle of the nineteenth century, pregnancy was an ambiguous condition, one that doctors wrote of continually as difficult to ascertain because of the deceptive nature of women's bodies.

Numerous Western physicians included false conceptions in their teaching texts on reproduction. Brudenell Exton, man-midwife at the Middlesex Hospital (Britain's first maternity hospital), perhaps most clearly defined this condition when he wrote in 1751: "there are two kinds of conception; the one where there is a foetus in the womb, which is called true; the other where there is a fleshy substance, which is called a mole, or any other strange body, from the morbid state of the uterus, which is termed false." Exton explained that a false conception or mole could closely mimic a true pregnancy and could fool the woman herself. However, Exton, as a trained physician, assured his students that he could discern the important differences, such as how, in the case of false conception, the breasts filled with serum instead of milk.[9]

In their medical texts and published articles, doctors differed on the origin of false conception. Some claimed it arose from corrupt conceptions, or the conjunction of two seeds gone awry. Others argued that it was the result of an embryo that died, but remained in the uterus and solidified. Still others maintained that false conceptions were merely coagulated blood. While they disagreed about the cause, physicians generally agreed on the existence, both theoretically and materially, of false conceptions.[10]

However, male doctors, who had little experience of the internal workings (or sensations) of the female body, were not the only ones to believe in this idea. Gender did not dictate theories of uterine actions. In other words, male physicians did not cling to the category of false conception merely because they did not possess the means to become pregnant themselves. This category was useful professionally for female practitioners as well. In her famous lectures, Madame du Coudray, royal midwife to the court of Louis XV of France, discussed "a chaos with no mark of a child," which resulted from a supposed pregnancy.[11] Doctors, midwives, and pregnant women agreed that the womb was a misleading organ and a site for the production and growth of numerous objects.

An important context for the ambiguity of eighteenth- and early nineteenth-century reproduction was the difficulty in positively determining pregnancy. Women could report breast tenderness, nausea, missing their "menses," or a growing belly, but these were all symptoms of a variety of illnesses at the time as well. These were also internal signs that were felt only by a woman and thus within the realm of female expertise. Male physicians could not diagnose nausea, and they were probably loath to press for proof of menstruation. Instead, physicians relied upon quickening, the first motions of the fetus within the womb (typically first felt by a woman sometime in the fourth month of pregnancy), as the most definitive sign of pregnancy. Numerous early modern medical experts emphasized the importance of quickening in pregnancy determination.[12] The influential German physician Wilhelm Gottfried Ploucquet claimed, "The movements of the fruit [fetus], in as much as they can be felt by an outsider or when they can be seen from the outside and are visible to an examiner, are one of the most privileged signs of pregnancy." Ploucquet valued the physical sensation of quickening as proof of pregnancy perhaps because it was an external sign that physicians could detect. Often a woman herself can feel quickening before it is discernible to others. For Ploucquet, quickening served as proof of pregnancy not when felt by women, but when determined by physicians. Like Abigail Adams's doctor, Ploucquet privileged the experienced sensations of the male medical expert over the experienced sensations of the pregnant woman.[13] Even motion felt by outsiders, however, could be a misleading symptom, as gastrointestinal movements could mimic quickening. But as many physicians highlighted, false conceptions could not move on their own, and thus quickening served as proof that other pregnancy symptoms were not the result of a mole.[14]

Prevailing philosophical understandings of pregnancy also played a role in shaping these medical and popular discussions about the uncertainty of pregnancy. For centuries natural philosophers had debated and investigated the development of a human being, a complex organism derived from the simplistic materials of sperm and ovum, with some historians tracing embryology back to the ancient Greeks.[15] In the late seventeenth century, the older theory of epigenesis—that organization developed from unorganized matter—fell out of favor because of its atheistic undertones. If God had created all of life at the beginning of time, then the formation of flesh and life where there had not been flesh and life before clearly contradicted church doctrine. The rival theory at the time, preformation, claimed that all adult structures were present—in the egg or sperm, depending on whom you asked—from the very beginning of development, and all the embryo needed to do during pregnancy was increase in size. As detailed by one historian, because the poor resolution of eighteenth-century microscope technology revealed neither preformed nor unformed beings in a fertilized egg, preformation represented "the triumph of reason over our limited sensation," thus fitting nicely within Enlightenment scientific ideals.[16] To be sure, there were problems with preformation, such as the nagging question: if God had made all these perfect individuals at the beginning of time, where did monsters come from? But it remained popular among scholars for much of the next hundred years.[17] Key to the understanding of eighteenth-century pregnancy was that under the theory of preformation, tissues expelled by a woman early in pregnancy that did not resemble a fully formed, but miniature, baby should be understood as bubbly lots or useless beings. A true pregnancy, after all, would produce an object that clearly resembled an infant, at any stage of the nine months. This conceptual framework allowed physicians and the lay public to interpret miscarriage tissues in a wide variety of ways.

Perhaps the most esteemed European medical expert on pregnancy and childbirth in the seventeenth and eighteenth centuries was the French obstetrician Francois Mauriceau. By the early eighteenth century, his influential text, translated into English as *The Diseases of Women with Child*, stood as the definitive midwifery text for any man purporting to be a scientifically trained physician. Agreeing with most learned medical men of the time, Mauriceau differentiated between true conception, "to which succeeds the Generation of the Infant in the Womb," and false conception, "which we may say is wholly against Nature, and there the Seeds change into Water, false Conceptions, Moles, or other strange Matter."[18] He further lectured on how to tell the difference between true and false "Great-Bellies," such as how a woman might believe herself pregnant if her breasts fill with milk, when it may in fact be whey in her breasts—a sure sign of a false "Great Belly."[19]

When it came to the premature ending of a pregnancy, however, Mauriceau's explanations become much more complex. He delineated the loss of a pregnancy between the first and the eighth day after conception as a "slip" because "at this time, there is nothing formed or figured, neither have the Seeds yet any firm Consistence, which is the Cause why it slips away so easily with the least opening of the Womb." From the first week to the second month, most expulsions were false conceptions, "which turn to Moles, if they continue any longer in the Womb." It is only after the third month that a practitioner would expect to see a fetus "wholly formed and animated," and thus such an expulsion should be labeled an "abortion."[20] Mauriceau left no room for the expulsion of a normally developing fetus prior to the third month—when such a normal fetus (by modern standards) certainly would more resemble an animal or an "inarticulate piece of flesh," than a human infant. Like many Western medical scholars of the time, he fit his clinical experience within the prevailing developmental theory of preformation. If what he saw in miscarriage cases did not appear infant-like, as most likely most early pregnancy losses would, then he interpreted them as false conceptions. Thus miscarriage, at least in the first few months, became defined as the expulsion of only false conceptions. French physician Pierre Dionis agreed in his 1719 text on midwifery, which established miscarriage as when a woman delivered "a false Conception, a Mole, or any extraneous Body form'd [sic] in the Womb."[21]

The uncertainty of premodern pregnancy loss derived not only from the difficulty of determining the variety of nonhuman objects that resulted from the event, but also from the difficulty in determining if the event had taken place at all. Because of the ambiguity inherent in pregnancy at the time (were a woman's breasts filling with milk or serum?), if she seemed to pass only clots of blood, physicians, midwives, and miscarrying women struggled to distinguish between loss of pregnancy or delayed menstruation, which created both a linguistic and conceptual slippage. Cessation of menstruation could easily fit in either category of pregnancy or illness due to any number of causes. Indeed, many women sought out therapies (such as tansy tea) to "bring on the menses" because they assumed they were ill and worried that illness would prevent pregnancy. Of course, it is quite possible (or probable) that other women used tansy tea to bring on the menses because they wanted to terminate a suspected pregnancy.[22] In the eighteenth century, indeed prior to the 1930s, the boundary dividing menstruation and early pregnancy loss was quite porous and far from stable. Doctors and families found pregnancy a condition that was difficult to discern, easily mistaken for another condition, and deceiving to all.

Meanwhile, eighteenth-century male physicians, seeking to expand their business into the realm of childbirth, were able to use this supposed falseness of the female body to their advantage. Male doctors had been writing of the "secrets of women," and how women's networks had kept those secrets tightly secure from prying male eyes, for many centuries. In the fourteenth century, changes in medical practice and education (such as the rise of the university) allowed more male practitioners to intrude upon traditional areas of female expertise—including pregnancy and childbirth. Gynecological texts that emerged from this movement often relied on the language of secrets and mysteries, suggesting that the female womb and the female practitioner were naturally deceptive, obstacles male physicians needed to overcome with the unveiling powers of science.[23] Male physicians also encountered resistance in their motions toward penetrating the traditionally female-controlled space of childbirth and other women's life-cycle events. Thus "secrets of women" took on a secondary meaning of knowledge retained within networks of women and kept out of reach of male scholars.[24]

This language of secrets and struggle between the man-midwife and the traditional female practitioner is clear in eighteenth-century medical writings as well. Many scholars claimed that not only should male doctors regard the signs of women's bodies with suspicion, but they should also distrust women's words, including those of female midwives. In his 1784 text, Irish obstetrician

Fielding Ould warned his fellow practitioners of the duplicitous nature of women. He claimed that in most cases, a false conception could be ruled out around the fourth month with the appearance of fetal motion, or quickening, but this was not an absolute rule. Ould recalled one case in which his patient insisted she felt the child moving, but when he reached into her uterus to help the delivery along, he found "a soft fleshy substance." Ould concluded, "this just serves to shew [sic], how little the mother's account is to be depended on in matters of this kind.[25] Ould presented his male expertise as far superior to any female kind. Women, he contended, whether midwives or pregnant females, could not understand the truth of the female body, and thus they should never be trusted on that subject.

She Was Mistaken: Women's Writings about Pregnancy

While Western doctors wrote about the useless beings produced by the mysterious cavern of the uterus, women also regularly discussed pregnancy in terms of ambiguity, uncertainty, and false alarms. Although there are not clear links between academic discussions about preformation, medical descriptions of fleshy morsels, and women's personal writings about the uncertainty of pregnancy, these three sources should be considered together as part of a larger culture that saw women's wombs as confusing and human development as a mystery.

From 1766 to 1791, Lady Mary Campbell Coke kept a diary detailing Georgian court life in London. Not much escaped Lady Coke's eye, or her pen. One of her interests proved to be the reproductive activities of British nobility. In her almost thirty years of writing, Coke included over one hundred references to who was pregnant, who might have been pregnant, and who was proven not to be pregnant. While at a time when physicians claimed that determining a "true" pregnancy was a complicated enterprise, and not one that should be left to mere women, the women in Coke's diary showed little hesitation in making such calls, but they, too, were often mistaken.

Typically, Lady Coke launched into the day's news by detailing the weather, the latest gossip, and pregnancy updates. In March 1768, Coke speculated on the reproductive activities of the Duchess of Buccleigh—"many people think that she will have two children; She certainly is uncommonly big,"—and proceeded to detail the latest scandal: "One of my servants had heard the most ridiculous story that ever was; that Lady Susan Steward had the day before owned her marriage with Lord Bute's second son, that she was married four years ago in Scotland." After remarking on her visit for the day, Coke came to the topic of Lady Burghersh, who had recently come to town and was thought to be "in a bad way." "When she came to town she was believed to be with child, but it proves a bad state of health," Coke recorded. This small snippet illustrates how early pregnancy could be a matter of public speculation, while also a mistaken supposition.[26]

For the next many years, Coke remained busy with her social reports and speculation. In 1774, Coke recorded the story of Madame D'Artois, who in April had hopes of being with child, only to watch those hopes "vanish." The following December, D'Artois again had hopes, but as Coke remarked, "'tis hoped Madame D'Artois is really with Child, but as it was twice before suspected, & proved a mistake, it is not yet publikly [sic] declared."[27] Pregnancy, at least among the aristocracy of Europe, was a subject open to public interpretation and scrutiny. But at the same time, it was a determination with which many women had difficulty. A public used to speculating about the reproductive activities of the ruling classes, an important subject for the economic and political well-being of many citizens, easily embraced the idea that women's bodies could be fickle and deceptive. Physicians attempting to gain professional legitimacy were not the only ones writing about the ambiguity of pregnancy; women like Lady Coke openly espoused the notion as well.

Lady Mary Coke was not the only woman chronicling the reproductive activities of eighteenth-century British royalty and aristocracy. Mary Clavering Cowper, Lady of the Bedchamber to the Princess of Wales in the early 1700s, also recorded multiple cases of pregnancies, supposed pregnancies, and deceptive bodies. Cowper reported of one woman who "fancies herself with child," and a neighbor who "reckons herself with child."[28] The language women such as Coke and Cowper used reflects a broader social understanding that pregnancy was difficult to discern, by medical and lay Europeans alike.

While physicians like Fielding Ould stressed the deceptive nature of women's bodies when it came to pregnancy and the superiority of medical expertise in such cases, many families discovered that even doctors could be mistaken. In 1685, Edward Conway wrote to his brother-in-law: "we have thoughts oftentimes in my wife's sickness, perhaps she may be breeding; but the excessive increase of her distemper, with many other reasons, so interrupted it, that they served only to torment." When they visited "the best doctors," Conway and his wife were assured that she was not pregnant. Mrs. Conway gave birth five months later.[29]

This cultural ambiguity surrounding pregnancy was not confined to the European continent, but shared by American doctors and families as well. In 1807, successful lecturer and physician Dr. Samuel Bard recorded his teachings on midwifery in one of the first American obstetrical texts. By 1819, the book was in its fifth edition and proved to be popular, probably most popular among students of medicine to whom Bard directed his book. In his chapter on diseases of women in "child-bed," Bard ended with a discussion of false conceptions. He warned his students that multiple objects could reside within a woman's womb and noted "the difficulty or rather impossibility of discovering their existence before their discharge."[30]

I Knew Better than He: Miscarriage and Bodily Expertise

While the idea of false conceptions and the deception of the reproducing female body was undoubtedly supported by medical and personal experiences with tumors, cysts, and other abdominal growths, miscarriage also served to prove the possibility of moles and fruits in eighteenth-century medicine. In the seventeenth and eighteenth centuries, European physicians were largely working within a philosophical framework for human development that portrayed most miscarriages as a result of false conception. In cases of conception gone wrong, they argued, nature stepped in and provided the fix by terminating the pregnancy. On the surface, the argument presented by eighteenth-century physicians to explain miscarriage should not sound all that foreign to our modern ears: miscarriage is the natural bodily process of getting rid of a pregnancy that is not normal or healthy. The hugely popular modern pregnancy guide, *What to Expect When You're Expecting*, attributes miscarriage to chromosomal or genetic defects or inadequate supplies of hormones; in effect, it is the body getting rid of a pregnancy gone awry.[31] But in the eighteenth century it was not so much that the pregnancy had gone awry, but rather that the pregnancy had not even commenced in the first place, because a true conception had never occurred. Instead of writing about genes and hormones, premodern physicians instead described a wide and fascinating array of objects that a womb could house and subsequently should expel.

Although natural philosophers and scholars began to lean away from preformation beginning in the middle of the 1700s, one legacy of this short-lived theory of human generation proved to be the idea that in normal pregnancies, the gestating child inside should always resemble a human. While Mauriceau himself described the process of conception and development in vague and abstract terms (neither clearly supporting preformation nor epigenesis), he did continue the tradition of false conceptions. As physicians like Mauriceau, Exton, and the American Samuel Bard attended women who were bleeding and experiencing labor pains early in pregnancy, they often interpreted the expelled tissues as nonhuman, and thus a pregnancy that was never going to work. The predominance of false conception helped physicians to view miscarriage, or the expulsion of materials from the uterus, as nature's fix to a misguided pregnancy.

If doctors and women understood true pregnancy to create something that looked like a miniature full-term infant, then a miscarriage of such a pregnancy would produce such a body. When doctors attended miscarriage cases, especially in the early stages of a woman's pregnancy, they often came across masses that did not possess the proper human structures. These encounters encouraged the idea that miscarriage was more common in cases of false conceptions. In his wildly popular (in both Britain and the United States) advice book, *Domestic Medicine*, British physician William Buchan informed his readers that miscarriages occurring in the first month were most likely false conceptions.[32]

If women experiencing early miscarriages most likely were carrying false conceptions to begin with, then doctors could more easily view pregnancy loss as nature's fix to a pernicious problem. Each report of the passage of clots, fleshy morsels, or useless beings lent credence to the idea that nature often took care of problem pregnancies via the mechanism of miscarriage. Doctors, therefore, did not need to spend much time or energy seeking to decrease miscarriage, for they would only then be acting against nature, which, in the eighteenth century, was never a good idea.

What, then, was the role of the physician in miscarriage? If we return to the story of Abigail Adams's miscarriage, it would seem that the physician's role was to show up, perhaps comfort the patient, but in the end he would have no useful knowledge about the event. Some of this impotence was surely due to the status of professional medicine in the newly emerging United States. While many English doctors in the colonies sought to replicate the medical system of Britain, such a class-based, Old-World organization appealed much less to many colonists. In Britain in the second half of the eighteenth century, medicine was a status profession; only upper-class gentlemen could attend medical school and as a result could practice true "learned" medicine. By this time, it was also a fairly old, well-established profession in Britain and many countries in Europe. In the colonies and eventually the United States, professional medicine was, not surprisingly, more democratic, and based more on one's ability to treat patients, rather than one's pedigree.[33]

The first medical school in the colonies was founded in Philadelphia in 1765, and the few schools established in the next three decades produced a very small number of university-educated practitioners. This shortage, however, did not alarm the public or the government, because the American medical marketplace in its early days was crowded with a variety of practitioners. Essentially, if men or women wanted to make a living in health care in the late eighteenth century, all they needed to do was start marketing themselves to their neighbors as having some sort of expertise in herbal remedies, wound stitching, childbirth, or any of the ills of early Americans. When Abigail Adams wrote to her husband, "I cannot say I have had any reason to alter my mind," she was thinking of medicine as an American, rather than as a former British subject. The physician, while deemed somewhat necessary in the event of a pregnancy producing "fits" and bleeding, could offer no real knowledge on what was happening inside of Adams's body, leaving her to rely on her own bodily expertise.

Fifty years later and thousands of miles away, another American woman shared Adams's frustrations with the ineptitude of medicine in the case of miscarriage. In 1816, Lucretia Orne Peabody married Alexander H. Everett and soon found herself living in a world of international politics and courtly manners. Alexander Everett, who served as a foreign diplomat for most of his professional life, whisked his bride all over Europe for decades, taking a final position as commissioner of China before his death there in 1847. The daughter of a wealthy and influential New Hampshire judge, Lucretia Everett may have been well prepared for the lifestyle awaiting her upon her marriage.[34] While overseas, Everett regularly corresponded with family members, perhaps most intimately with her husband's sister, Sarah Everett Hale, who lived in Boston. The letters from Everett to Hale are rich with stories about the cultures, fashions, and people Everett encountered and enjoyed, and they provide fascinating details, such as her feelings of awkwardness at being presented at various European courts.

In August 1820, while residing at The Hague, Everett wrote to Hale about her health. Not wanting to trouble her sister-in-law, Everett wrote, "You complain that I do not mention myself more particularly but it is because I have nothing agreeable to tell you and don't like to write of my own afflictions." Nonetheless, Everett did end up describing one affliction—a recent pregnancy loss. She recounted, "When I wrote to you in February, my health was perfectly good and I had more reason to hope than I have ever had before that I should have a living child in May—but a few days afterward I perceived the usual symptoms of premature birth." Nearly six months pregnant, Everett determined that her pregnancy was over. After only four years of marriage, Everett was not only childless but was also experienced enough with miscarriage to be able to detect the "usual" signs.[35]

As a woman of high status in a European country, Everett followed common practice and called in a physician to consult with about the miscarriage. As she described later, he insisted that "there was no change ... and that it was nerves, that [she] must go more into company and mix more in the gaieties of society to keep off melancholy." Everett was not pleased with his diagnosis and recommendations and reminded Hale, "I knew from similar circumstances better than he." The following month she proved to her doctors that she did know better by delivering the products of her miscarriage. She closed the account with the remark: "I am almost discouraged now that I have had so many misfortunes of that kind, except when I am in the family way and then hope always prevails over fear."[36]

Three years later, Everett again expressed her sadness and frustration over a miscarriage and medical "expertise." This time writing from Brussels, she reported to Hale that letters from home came at an ideal time, when she "was needing all the consolations of friends," because Everett had again lost a pregnancy, what she had taken to calling "the same unhappy circumstances that have marked all my former ones." This time it was perhaps more deeply disappointing because Everett had been taking a course of medicine that had raised her hopes even more. Once again, her medical advisors proved incompetent: "From the time I was conscious that I had nothing more to hope until my confinement a period of six weeks my physician and accoucheur visited me constantly and never could discover the least change in bodily health and therefore could not administer any remedy from not knowing what complaint they had to treat and they were perfectly convinced that I should be happily confined at the proper period." Everett ended her tragic story by divulging, "I cannot tell you how sad it is to be lingering for so long a time conscious that there is no remedy but patience."[37]

After this latest miscarriage, Everett's husband suggested seeking out the advice of the "most skillful surgeon" in England to help her carry a child to full term. Everett's hopes were waning after seven years of numerous miscarriages, and she lamented: "I have but very little hope that any advice or medicine would be of any use."[38] While her social station dictated that she seek medical aid during her pregnancy, especially if that pregnancy was not proceeding properly, Everett had little confidence in that medical aid. Her doctors continually disregarded her bodily expertise even after her deliveries proved her correct again and again.

The two stories of Abigail Adams and Lucretia Everett represent the role of medicine in American miscarriage in the late eighteenth and early nineteenth centuries. For many women, there actually was no role for professional medicine. Doctors cost money, and probably most families saw little reason to use their paltry funds on a gentleman who would pat their heads and insist that nothing was amiss, even if a woman knew, as Everett did, that "all was going wrong." For Americans, calling instead for aid from a female relative or a female midwife or reading about miscarriages in books such as Buchan's *Domestic Medicine* was mostly likely the more common response to a miscarriage.

But in the late eighteenth and early nineteenth centuries, doctors were increasingly gaining entrance into women's bedrooms for reproductive issues, beginning with the upper classes.[39] We can use these clinical encounters to better understand why it took so long for doctors to gain any authority over the treatment or definition of miscarriage. Male doctors, like the one treating Lucretia Everett, relied upon external signs of the body as a way to differentiate their expertise of the female body from that of the pregnant woman. As Everett lamented, her physicians could not "discover the least change in bodily health," and thus they disregarded her fears that "all was going wrong."

Such encounters left women like Lucretia Everett and Abigail Adams unsatisfied with doctors and the medical wisdom concerning miscarriage. Still living in a culture that largely trusted female authority when it came to childbirth (midwives delivered around 80 percent of all babies in the United States in 1800), these women resisted the male physicians' impulse to redefine miscarriage and pregnancy as only sensible to their "educated" hands and eyes.[40] In the end, American physicians had little to offer in terms of prevention and treatment of miscarriage, or even knowledge of what was happening inside the female uterus. Prior to the 1830s, a clinical encounter in a case of miscarriage was more likely to result in women and families doubting that there was any place for a male physician rather than seeing it as a meaningful step in the medical authority over miscarriage.

3

Before Its Due Time

Setting Standards in Miscarriage, 1830–1860s

Amelia Ryerse Harris became an avid diary-keeper in her later life. Starting her personal writings at the age of fifty-nine, Harris devotedly detailed the many social gatherings she hosted as well as the health and news of her ten children and their families. In 1865, one of those events suitable for recording in her diary was a miscarriage suffered by her daughter, Amelia Harris Griffin. On May 10, 1865, Harris devoted an entry to her daughter: "Yesterday all day Amelia was ailing and confined herself to the sofa. She felt so weak that she felt she had better go to bed before her visitors arrived." Griffin's illness soon became apparent, as "she had scarcely got into her room before symptoms of a miscarriage appeared. The Doctor (Landor) was sent for but his skill could not prevent the misfortune."[1]

Harris continued the entry, which followed Griffin's condition the next day. She reported: "She looks very weak but I hope with care will soon gain strength." Some of Griffin's weakness, Harris supposed, derived from the miscarriage coming so soon after a difficult childbirth, two reproductive struggles that might send Griffin "into a decline." Harris described the miscarriage as a misfortune but was quick to add: "but if the misfortune ends here we shall have great reason to be thankful." Griffin, unlike Mary Longfellow, survived her miscarriage to live another fifty-three years. But her miscarriage proved to be a long illness, requiring medical attention and months of careful care.[2]

For some women, miscarriage in nineteenth-century America resulted in prolonged ill health or was even fatal. Often, families like the Longfellows and the Griffins saw a clear need for medical aid in the face of high fevers, severe hemorrhaging, loss of consciousness, or other harrowing symptoms. And by the 1830s, American physicians began to show interest in how they might be specially equipped to handle such cases. Influenced by new philosophical and scientific understandings of pregnancy, doctors began to reframe their interpretations of miscarriage. Rather than holding to older views that miscarriage was nature's way of getting rid of a false conception, medical elites instead began describing miscarriage as a problem, and one that only they had the knowledge to solve. By refashioning miscarriage as serious and risky, as well as a phenomenon best understood by the science of medicine, physicians attempted to convince the American public to look to them for aid with this reproductive calamity. A survey of publications by physicians from 1830 through the 1860s reveals a dramatic increase in the number of discussions about miscarriage, and an apparent increase of miscarriage cases that regular doctors attended, which could illustrate the success of medical authority over miscarriage. But a deeper study, especially into how women viewed these new medical leanings, shows that American physicians had little to offer potential patients in terms of explanation, prevention, or treatment of pregnancy loss. It was almost as if doctors began to recognize the potential value of their entry into miscarriage cases, but they could not decide, or perhaps not agree upon, how to convince miscarrying women to invite them in.

In medical texts and popular health guides from the 1830s through the 1860s, physicians and health writers typically focused on three aspects of miscarriage: a definition, lengthy lists of causes, and proposed courses of action. Taken alone, these emerging medical narratives of miscarriage could point to increased patient interest in the medical management of pregnancy loss. However, throughout this time, women continued to express frustration at the lack of medical capabilities, and instead they sought to understand the experience outside of medical definitions or interpretations, much as Abigail Adams and Lucretia Everett had done decades before. It would take a lot more than a doctor's proclamation before most American women saw value in medical miscarriage "expertise."

Definition: Epigenesis and the Shifting Meaning of Miscarriage

By the turn of the nineteenth century, distrust of women's expertise about their own bodies remained a key aspect of professionalizing physicians, especially for doctors involved in the competition for business with female midwives, but doctors also began to leave behind the rhetoric of the mystery of pregnancy. Influenced by philosophical, cultural, and medical shifts, physicians instead began to focus on a particular and universal object contained within pregnancy and lost via miscarriage. Thus by the 1830s and 1840s, gone were the descriptions of indeterminate flesh and fruits that could grow in wombs, and in their place arose the notion of a standardized fetus, present in all pregnancies.

The first thing to go was the idea of false conception. In 1807, Thomas Denman, a former naval surgeon who had shifted to midwifery after attending lectures of the great Scottish obstetrician William Smellie, argued that, although other practitioners believed in false conceptions as akin to monstrous births, he regarded such amorphous tissues as products of true conceptions: "For though it has the appearance of a shapeless mass of flesh, if examined carefully with a knife, various parts of the child may be discovered, lying together, in apparent confusion, but in actual regularity."[3] Rather than being deceived by the apparent confusion of the fleshy substance that might result from a miscarriage, Denman presented the idea that hidden within such visual chaos was the natural order of human development. This new interpretation represents a major modification in the medical response to the products of miscarriage. Under the theory of preformation, doctors understood ambiguous materials as the confusion of a false conception, a nonhuman being produced by a disordered female body. But in the early 1800s, physicians began to interpret apparent disorganization instead as merely obscuring the true order in nature, but order that could be detected only by a properly medically trained eye.

This shift away from false conception was the result of an intersection of broader social and cultural moves that acted together to bring doctors in closer and more consistent contact with pregnant women and their miscarried fetuses. The increasing popularity of epigenesis, however, recast what those miscarriage products could mean. In the 1740s, three scholars, French philosopher Pierre Louis Moreau de Maupertuis, French naturalist Georges Louis de Buffon, and English biologist John Turberville Needham, independently proposed epigenetic theories that offered a seemingly new view of generation. Epigenesis, the concept that highly organized matter arose from simplistic materials, at its core was not a new idea. In his *On the Generation of Animals*, considered by many historians to be the first systematic treatise on embryology, the ancient scholar Aristotle described the embryology of the chick, noting that not all structures were present at early stages: "And our failure to see them is not because they are too small." Aristotle described what he termed "epigenesis" (Greek translation is "upon generation"), or a succession of gradual changes to transform unorganized mass into the well-orchestrated collection of parts that became an adult.[4] Maupertuis, Buffon, and Needham utilized Aristotle's argument, agreeing that the various organs and structures apparent in a full-term infant developed over the course of the nine-month gestation and were not present at the time of conception. Not surprisingly, many eighteenth-century scholars resisted the notion of epigenesis, especially those seeking to preserve the religious foundations on which preformation rested.[5]

The reasons why scholars began to move away from preformation and support epigenesis toward the close of the eighteenth century are not entirely clear. One possibility lies in the new national interests in Europe concerning the pregnant body and the unborn being within. As European governments became more focused on generating a large and strong population as a generator of wealth, nations such as France and Britain invested in monitoring pregnancy and childbirth (to ensure more healthy citizens) through the creation of lying-in hospitals and the promotion of educated, scientific male midwives.[6] These changes, in turn, increased the opportunities for male scholars and physicians to come into contact with pregnant women and embryos, allowing them more chances to observe human development and how it might not fit easily within the theory of preformation. Some historians contend that the rise of physician support for the return to Hippocratic theories of generation in France and Britain, theories that lent themselves to epigenesis, was the deciding factor.[7] Others maintain that it was the more general shift in biological thought that emphasized teleological organization (physical organization based on intended purpose) in the natural world that led thinkers away from preformation.[8] Still others look to the work of particular biologists, especially those in German universities, as the instigation of this movement.[9]

While the popular move from preformation to epigenesis is more likely explained by a combination of all of the above factors, historians agree that this shift was largely complete by the end of the eighteenth century. Although this philosophical shift impacted the practice of childbirth in many Western countries and paved the way for the development of modern human embryology, it also created a new medical understanding of miscarriage. Under the theory of preformation, a true pregnancy (coming from a true conception) could only result in the expulsion of an object that was clearly human, and one that resembled a tiny, but fully formed, infant. When doctors, midwives, and families encountered a product of miscarriage that did not appear human, they could call on the explanation of false conception to account for this creature. Under epigenesis, however, odd-looking "creatures" (as some physicians dubbed them) were reclassified as the result of normal gestation. To recall the ideas of Thomas Denman, if one looked hard enough (or with the proper expertise), one should be able to discover the natural order in these seemingly unnatural beings. By the middle of the nineteenth century the category of false conception fell into obscurity (or was remanded to the category of outdated theories) because it was no longer needed. Physicians could now "see" normal human development in all types of strange clumps and clots.

Historians of science have long known that scientists bring assumptions, whether they be methodological or epistemological in nature, to knowledge production, and such was the case with miscarriage products.[10] American doctors' writings about miscarriage throughout the nineteenth century reveal these assumptions clearly. When the preformation theory was still supported, and continuing through a few decades after elite European scholars had abandoned the theory, physicians assumed that clots and indistinguishable tissues did not count as knowledge about normal development, and thus the bedside of a miscarrying woman was not viewed as a site for obtaining such knowledge. But beginning in the 1830s, the new way to "see" human development was to dig deeper into the clots and other masses that came out of pregnant women's vaginas.

The assumptions had shifted so dramatically that by 1854, prominent Scottish obstetrician J. Matthews Duncan could easily argue that false conceptions were extremely rare in humans, and he even advised his fellow doctors to consider cases of supposed false pregnancy as purposeful deceptions by their female patients.[11] In America, the story was much the same. Charles Meigs, one of the most influential obstetricians of the time, reformulated the category of "moles" from products of false conceptions to products of true conceptions that had died and remained within the womb.[12] This philosophical transformation in human development created a new venue for scientific knowledge (the bedside of the miscarrying woman) as well as a new specimen for which American physicians could hunt. And by the 1850s, plenty of these medical men were hot on the trail—ready to bring their expertise and rational order to the realm of pregnancy loss.

The shift from preformation to epigenesis not only invalidated the use of false conception as a category, but it also reshaped the definition of miscarriage. What was previously described as either an event that could include any number of objects (moles or bubbly lots to name two), or as only an event without notice of the object involved, now became a situation that was defined solely by the singular object involved. While eighteenth-century pregnancy loss was delineated as just that, the loss of a pregnancy, beginning in the 1830s doctors explained pregnancy loss as real only when it involved a particular object, and an increasingly universal object. As physicians looked to discover what they could about pregnancy and human development from cases of miscarriage, they became particularly focused on the embryo or fetus involved. American doctors looked to reformulate the phenomenon of miscarriage into a medical problem, and like many other nineteenth-century medical professionalization stories, a key aspect to this reformulation was to set standards and create rational order where there seemingly was once only chaos.

This focus on the object contained in pregnancy and lost in miscarriage was a new priority by the 1830s, and one rarely seen in the previous century. In his 1785 text, John Aitken defined miscarriage as "the separation of the placenta and chorion from the uterus, or the disease and death of the child."[13] Jean Astruc described it as the disengagement of the fetus from the "matrix," while Alexander Hamilton (the Scottish physician, not the first U.S. treasury secretary and current cultural icon) explained miscarriage as the dissolution of the connection between the child and parent.[14] Francois Mauriceau, perhaps the most influential European obstetric physician of the eighteenth century, described it as a "slipping away" and effluxion (the act of flowing out).[15] Most eighteenth-century physicians agreed that one should identify miscarriage based on the actions involved, or simply define it as the woman's pregnant state coming to an end.

Each of these men—Aitken, Hamilton, and Mauriceau—included his miscarriage definitions in a text geared toward elite males learning about midwifery. Both Aitken and Hamilton taught at the University of Edinburgh, considered by many to be the center of elite education and research on midwifery at the time. Mauriceau, who had a bustling business among the French aristocracy, addressed his book to "gentlemen" practicing the art of midwifery. In their definitions of miscarriage, each author envisioned a particular woman, the most common patient of his students: an upper-class woman of superior breeding and great gentility. Clinical encounters with such women probably did not include an internal examination or even much beyond a cursory glance at the miscarried tissues. Instead, the physician's job in such an encounter was to ensure the woman recovered sufficiently to endeavor to get pregnant again, and thus continue inheritance lines. The social role of European elite doctors, like Hamilton and his students, encouraged them to interpret miscarriage as merely a temporary termination in sustaining family lineage rather than anything akin to the emerging embryological studies on chickens. Elite women, after all, were not barnyard hens.

By the middle of the nineteenth century, in contrast, doctors' writings focused on the centrality of the object produced in their definitions of miscarriage, or rather, the uniform types of objects. The primary objects involved in miscarriage became far more ordered and regular than the motley assortment of things that had been believed a century earlier to come out of a woman's vagina. Chicago physician Edwin Hale illustrated this careful order in his four divisions of miscarriage: "(1) Ovular, when the ovum is lost before it is impregnated. (2) Embryonic, when the impregnated ovum is expelled before the placenta has formed its uterine attachment. (3) Foetal, when the expulsion occurs after the last date, and before the viability of the child; and (4) when the child is born capable of living, or viable, but before the end of normal pregnancy."[16] Rather than describing the separation or the disease involved, Hale defined miscarriage solely on the basis of which type of object a woman delivered.

While Hale included the birth of a viable child in his discussion of miscarriage, most nineteenth-century physicians regarded these "premature births" as a distinct category. The other three terms—ovum, embryo, and fetus—filled the medical literature as the key objects expelled by the female body. Generally, the use of the three was not quite as orderly as Hale's definition; most physicians relied on "fetus" to describe the tissues they encountered, saving "embryo" or "ovum" to highlight an especially small or early specimen.[17] This placement of a uniform object at the center of the definition of miscarriage quickly became standard in articles and teaching texts, reflecting the shifting ideas of what a pregnant woman held within her body, and thus expelled through miscarriage. While the description of a concrete object involved in miscarriage was not necessarily revolutionary, the narrowing of the groups of objects—from moles, animals, growths, and lots to fetus only—and the disappearance of more abstract artifacts—chaos, useless beings—imbued the event with scientific and medical underpinnings, especially since these were medically constructed categories. Uneducated midwives or even untrained mothers could label an object as gristle or a growth, but supposedly only doctors could properly identify an ovum. The attention on the object "expelled" by miscarriage, as so many described it, also provides clues to the shifting import of what physicians could take away from such cases. Physicians seemed less interested in miscarriage as the end of a pregnancy and more focused on it as a phenomenon that produced a material result.

Defining the Danger

Beginning in the 1840s, as medical articles reporting on miscarriage cases flourished and teaching texts expanded their sections on "abortion," physicians also sought to reinterpret miscarriage as inherently dangerous, and all cases of miscarriage as dangerous. Charles D. Meigs, perhaps the most well-known physician of midwifery in the United States in the middle of the nineteenth century, informed his students that miscarriage was among the most common and most "vexatious" of diseases and accidents of pregnancy and was often followed by "long years of broken health, and by weakness which is never fully recovered from."[18] In the 1873 printing of his clinical lectures, Gunning S. Bedford, professor of obstetrics at the University of New York, opened his lecture on abortion by labeling miscarriage as interesting for two reasons: it was frequent, and it involved the female in great danger.[19] Many others stressed the dangers of the severe blood loss that frequently accompanied miscarriage.[20]

The warnings of the hazards of miscarriage appeared with even more frequency in medical journal articles dealing with the subject. Doctors repeatedly described cases in which their female patients suffered grave symptoms of miscarriage. In 1854, A. I. Cummings described the difficulty new doctors facing miscarriage had because it was a case where "the vital fluid is flowing, not *guttatim*, but *in torrents*, as it were, and when immediate relief must be had—the flowing torrent be immediately checked or death will ensue."[21] John Holston recounted a case of a woman who had been hemorrhaging for three days before he attended her, and Horatio Wood chronicled a patient whom he found "lying in a cataleptic trance," because of miscarriage.[22]

Recording these frightening cases in the pages of medical journals perhaps helped physicians convince themselves of the need for medical care in cases of miscarriage, but talking among themselves in professional journals about the dangers of miscarriage got doctors only so far. Medical periodicals, such as *Medical and Surgical Reporter* or *Boston Medical and Surgical Journal*, served as forums for internal discussions among physicians who sought out the advice of colleagues, aimed to commiserate with fellow practitioners, or attempted to gain professional acclaim. These reports and articles, however, did little to increase the business of physicians. A doctor might have displayed an article in his clinic office or informed his patients of a recent publication, but throughout the nineteenth century, these accolades were not valued by most of the American public. The nineteenth-century medical marketplace was a crowded one, and physicians needed to utilize other venues for appealing to and convincing potential patients of their value.

If physicians could convince women and their families of the perils of miscarriage and paint themselves as the necessary saviors, they might gain further entry into the business, but medical journals were not the right venue for this. Instead, physicians needed to speak directly to women and families and scare them into calling a physician for every case of miscarriage. Doctors wanted to take this new medical reframing of miscarriage and utilize it to convince their patients that they, and only they, should be considered the ultimate authority on miscarriage, and the most appropriate venue for this was the domestic health guide.

The existence of the domestic health guide in America dates back to the colonial era, but in the 1840s, publishers focused on pamphlets and books aimed at women and particularly at women's health.[23] Readers flocked to domestic health guides as a result of multiple social forces that were at work in the first half of the nineteenth century. Changes in medicine and reading habits created a new space, and a new market, for these home-remedy manuals. In Jacksonian America, many citizens began to value self-reliance in all aspects of life, including medicine. By the 1830s, countless Americans who were frustrated with the ineffectual and brutal therapies that were common in medical treatments began to seek alternatives. Faced with the purging, puking, and bleeding of Benjamin Rush's heroic medicine that was so favored in the eighteenth century, many Americans were losing faith in "learned" medicine, especially when it came with a steep price tag. As a result, in the first half of the nineteenth century, regular physicians faced strong public opposition to their attempts at creating a monopoly over the field of health care.[24]

American patients not only sought out new types of practitioners, but they also made attempts to treat their ailments at home. Following the model promoted by Samuel Thomson (founder of the eponymous sect Thomsonian medicine), numerous Americans endeavored to become their own doctors, often with the help of patent medicines or local physiological groups.[25] One of the more geographically far-reaching developments in this new medical system was the domestic medical guide, whose popularity grew enormously over the course of the century. A number of these manuals went through multiple editions over many decades, and some even saw total sales in the millions.[26] By the 1840s, Americans could choose from a number of health manuals, such as the wildly popular encyclopedic *Gunn's Domestic Medicine* or the more focused work of Edward Dixon, *Woman and Her Diseases, from the Cradle to the Grave.*

Coinciding with the rise in domestic health guide publishing was a general increase in the number of readers nationwide. Throughout the first half of the nineteenth century, literacy rates rose among native-born whites, so that by 1850 90 percent reported that they could read.[27] Of course, we cannot assume readership was equally distributed over class and race, although the trend seemed to be fairly well distributed geographically; it was not merely an urban trend in the Northeast, as rural areas of New England, the Midwest, and the South showed similar new interest in health books as well.[28]

Literacy rates of women showed the sharpest increase. A distinctly female novel-reading public emerged in the first few decades of the nineteenth century, and this group began exploring other genres by the 1850s.[29] One of these genres was advice literature. Not only did more nineteenth-century women read than their mothers had, but also the scope of their reading broadened to include countless books on how to manage their families and their households. For the most part, domestic advice literature relied upon the newly literate white middle class as its audience, a growing and increasingly influential group at the time.[30]

From these popular and widely read books, we can glean how physicians constructed their arguments to the lay public for why miscarriage required medical interventions. One such argument was to convince their patients of the great danger posed by miscarriage, perhaps hoping that fear would lead to increased use of regular medicine. In 1843, Alfred Hall, a traveling botanical physician who practiced primarily on the East Coast, warned his readers that miscarriage "ought to be considered at all time exceedingly dangerous—both debilitating to the general health of the female and very injurious to the uterus."[31] John C. Gunn, perhaps the most popular physician dispensing advice at the time, agreed with that view in his home medical guide, citing miscarriage as a "severe trial to the maternal constitution," and P. C. Dunne followed suit, stating: "There cannot be a question that miscarriage . . . is productive of the most injurious and serious effects upon the female constitution."[32]

Perhaps the only writer to downplay the dangers of pregnancy loss was Dr. A. M. Mauriceau, who referred to himself as a professor of the diseases of women. In his 1860 book, *The Married Woman's Private Medical Companion*, he stressed that miscarriage was a subject "in respect to which there exists much misapprehension and ignorance, causing useless and unnecessary alarm." Instead, Mauriceau claimed that the dangers of abortion or miscarriage were exaggerated, and that most cases resulted in safe recoveries.[33] It is key to note, however, that Mauriceau may have been speaking from a conflict of interest. Historians have traced the writer of these texts (who notably chose the same last name of the famous and trusted eighteenth-century French obstetrician) to be either the brother or the husband of Madame Restelle, perhaps the most infamous abortion provider of the nineteenth century.[34] It would have benefited Restelle's business if a domestic health guide, authored by a learned physician, touted the safety of miscarriages—both accidental and induced.

A survey of medical periodicals shows numerous miscarriage case reports that reveal families often agreed with physicians—miscarriage could be dangerous and therefore required a doctor's presence. For most of these families, however, calling for a doctor's help was not necessary simply because a woman was miscarrying, but it was imperative when that miscarriage became dangerous with symptoms of severe or extended bleeding, pain, or other complications. In 1840, William Zollickoffer attended a Mrs. O., who was experiencing an extreme flooding of blood. She told Zollickoffer that she was afraid the bleeding would end her life before he could arrive.[35] In 1846, Thomas Osborne was called into a case in which the woman involved experienced pain and bleeding for four months.[36] Indeed, for some women, calling a doctor was the right choice not immediately upon determining a miscarriage, but when the symptoms continued past the delivery of a fetus, lasting days, weeks, or even months longer.

Framing miscarriage as dangerous seemed to be a usable strategy for doctors. It was not unusual for many families to appeal to physicians in cases of seemingly dangerous symptoms. However, doctors tried to use this custom to claim that *all* cases of miscarriage were dangerous or least could be if a doctor was not in attendance. The cases that appeared in medical journals show the ineffectiveness of this claim. In 1848, a family in Woodstock, Maine, called for the help of Dr. D. W. Davis. As he later described in an article for the *Boston Medical and Surgical Journal*, Mrs. C. did not call for medical aid on suspecting a miscarriage or even on experiencing a miscarriage. Mrs. C. sought out Dr. Davis four weeks after delivering a three-month fetus because she had continued to bleed ever since, and the "discharge had become copious and extremely offensive." Like many families, the C's continued to see miscarriage as a domestic concern; it was only copious bleeding that was a medical concern.[37]

Anything and Everything: The Causes of Miscarriage

While they were busy presenting cases illustrating the danger and need for medical attention in cases of miscarriage, American physicians also sought new explanations for why this fearsome event attacked women, and seemingly so many women. In teaching texts doctors began compiling long lists of pregnancy-loss causes, including a vast array of daily activities, behaviors, and even emotions. Although physicians did not neglect miscarriage causes in medical texts prior to 1830, their discussions were short, vague, and focused primarily on the death of the fetus as a cause. By the 1840s and 1850s, medical writings on miscarriage causation expanded to include long lists of social pursuits, environmental aspects, and anatomical conditions.

In the first half of the nineteenth century, physicians referred to only a few causes of miscarriage. Samuel Bard's 1819 publication, *A Compendium of the Theory and Practice of Midwifery*, which briefly stated that fatigue, exercise, shocks, and frequent sexual intercourse could be dangerous for a pregnant woman, noted that the explicit cause of miscarriage was simple: "the death of the foetus; a separation of the ovum from the womb; [and] the cessation of the healthy action of gestation."[38] In essence, miscarriage was caused by the pregnancy no longer progressing as nature intended. Bard's short musings on causation imply that he saw no reason to investigate further into why a woman miscarried—perhaps because he still viewed miscarriage as a natural fix to an unnatural pregnancy.

But physicians soon relied instead on lengthy lists in their nineteenth-century medical texts. In his 1841 text, Edward Rigby informed his students that "premature expulsion may be induced by a great variety of causes," and he proceeded to include general debility, dyspepsia, depressing passions of the mind, insufficient nourishment, toothache, blows, lifting heavy weights, inflammation of the vagina or bladder, too frequent sexual intercourse, and "the mere act of walking," among them.[39] A look through medical texts of the second half of the nineteenth century reveals an impressive display of activities, conditions, emotions, and illnesses that health writers thought caused pregnancy loss. In 1853, Thomas Cock, a physician at the New York Lying-In Asylum, published a manual of obstetrics. In the section on miscarriage, Cock found so many possible causes that he divided them into eight categories: ovuline, uterine, constitutional, mechanical, medicines, emotional, and assigned. The first category included different conditions of the ovum or placenta, such as a fatty placenta, rupture of umbilical vein, and plurality of ova. In the second category, he described a variety of uterine conditions and positions as well as cancer, tumors, placenta previa, and dysmenorrhoea.[40] Constitutional causes encompassed a number of diseases including syphilis, tuberculosis, dysentery, constipation, piles, as well as women who may be "advanced in life," or phthisical.[41] The category of mechanical causes consisted of sexual intercourse, violent exercise ("as horseback, jolting over rough roads"), blows, falls, vomiting, dancing, hysteria, epilepsy, and operations. After listing medicines that he thought could lead to pregnancy loss, and including "terror, &c.," under emotional causes, Cock closed with his "assigned causes" of odors, sights, laughter, crying, itching, sneezing, hot rooms, and hot baths.[42]

In 1864, Hugh Hodge advised that a dead ovum, falls, swellings, tight dresses, mental afflictions, violent passions, inordinate sexual excitement, disgusting tastes, intestinal irritants, and hemorrhoids could all lead to a loss of pregnancy.[43] The lists of causes seemed to grow only as physicians grew more and more interested in the medical possibilities of miscarriage, so that by the 1870s, Alexander Milne could create one of the longer lists, and among his almost seventy distinct causes he included: hemorrhoids, cancer, fissure of the rectum, drastic cathartics, fecal worms, bladder stones, lactation, the pain and shock of tooth extraction, syphilis, excessive sexual intercourse, ovarian disease, gastric irritation, chronic vomiting, coughing, sneezing, scrofula, debility, lead poisoning, anemia, smallpox, fever, morbid state of the placenta, falls, blows, overexertion, jumping, riding, lifting heavy loads, excessive joy, grief, rage, sorrows of captivity, and apprehension of death.[44]

Beginning in the 1840s and continuing throughout the rest of the century, physicians also often included very general causes, in essence constructing categories into which an almost endless array of events, conditions, or habits could fit. Like Cock, some doctors referred to "odors" and "sights" as causes of pregnancy loss, without offering any further qualification of what type.[45] Others added that "general health" could be an important factor in the safety of the pregnancy, while D. Berry Hart included "general debility."[46] In 1875, William Leishman simply mentioned "accidents" among his causes, leaving room for any number of specific major or minor accidents and perhaps little ease in the minds of his patients.[47] Most of the teaching texts I surveyed seemed to support the words of J. K. Shirk, who in his 1884 text simply stated the causes as "an almost endless number and variety."[48]

By the late 1840s, the lists of the causes of miscarriage also began to include more scientific-sounding anatomical abnormalities. In 1848, William Tyler Smith claimed that fatty degeneration of the chorion and placenta could lead to pregnancy loss, while

Gunning Bedford included malposition of the uterus on his 1861 list of causes.[49] This trend continued as physicians looked to "pathological conditions of the maternal organism," and structural conditions of the uterus as important causes to note.[50] The increase in anatomical and "scientific" causes of miscarriage in these lists may also point to physicians' interest in finding causes that could be determined only by scientific experts, such as themselves, as another avenue for professional authority.

One of the most apparent patterns in doctors' warnings about what could lead to a loss of pregnancy was the language of excess. Throughout the prophylactic literature, these American doctors highlighted the risks involved in living to extremes of some sort. In these sections, doctors counseled each other to have the patient avoid excess and violence in a number of activities and states of mind.[51] Physicians also often included advice about rest, quiet, and calm in body and mind in order to prevent pregnancy loss. Fleetwood Churchill recommended a light diet; William Playfair called for general rest; and A. S. Church advocated quieting nervous fears and remaining in a recumbent position.[52] In 1860, Thomas Tanner counseled that "everything should be done to insure tranquility of mind and body," and he proceeded to advise on diet, regularity of bowels, exercise, and the use of a mattress rather than a featherbed for sleeping.[53] Edward Rigby contended: "the mere act of walking, when carried to such an extent as to induce exhaustion, will suffice," to induce a miscarriage.[54]

Hidden from these authoritative-sounding lists of all the numerous activities, behaviors, and mindsets that could cause a miscarriage in the texts that physicians wrote in order to train the next generation was the origins of these causes. Doctors did not develop the connection between violent emotions, sudden frights, or falls and losing a pregnancy in a laboratory, nor did they derive the link between a healthy pregnancy and walking slowly from complex theories of the physiology of pregnancy. Instead, these causes, as revealed by case reports, came from the stories women told their doctors during the event of a miscarriage. Pregnant and miscarrying women played key roles in the development of medical theory.

In 1852, A. W. Barrows of Hartford, Connecticut, was called in to see Mrs. J., who was suffering labor pains in her fourth or fifth month of pregnancy. In his write-up of the case in the *American Journal of the Medical Sciences*, Barrows reported that his patient had attributed her condition to "over-exertion, particularly in washing windows, when she was obliged to reach."[55] Barrows took his patient's evaluation at face value and recorded it without further commentary, indicating that he either believed her overexertion to be a true cause, or he at least believed such a cause was possible.

Other physicians documented causes provided by their patients, adding little medical input to these determinations. In 1861, Dr. Horatio Wood attended a twenty-one-year-old woman in a cataleptic trance during her sixth month of pregnancy. In his article Wood described that upon inquiry (of whom he did not divulge), "it was ascertained that she had had a violent quarrel, which had caused her present condition."[56] In these clinical encounters, the cause of pregnancy loss seemed to have followed a straight path from a woman's or family's oral account to a doctor's published report. In 1867, Dr. Markoe was called in to attend a woman who was four months pregnant. She informed Markoe that her pregnancy had been progressing well, and she had even felt movement, when disaster struck. Upon returning home from a social gathering, "she was thrown somewhat gently from the carriage, and considerably alarmed. On reaching home, she observed that at the very moment of the accident, all the symptoms which had been going on so favorably, had suddenly ceased." Upon his examination, Markoe agreed with the woman that her fetus had died, and he helped her through its delivery four months later. This woman had ascertained not only that a loss of pregnancy was imminent, but also that her accident and alarm were the chief causes. Markoe seemingly agreed with her, and he reported her assertions at a meeting of the New York Pathological Society.[57]

The case reported by Ohio physician J. Stolz in 1866 reveals that for some women, there was a very important reason to provide a cause for their miscarriage. Stolz was called in to aid "a young woman of but sixteen, lately married, and in much pain and distress." When Stolz asked his patient why she might be losing her pregnancy, she recounted that she had fallen the previous evening and had been in pain ever since. When the woman refused the treatment Stolz recommended to prevent a miscarriage, Stolz became suspicious and continued questioning her. Stolz wrote that the young woman finally disclosed that "she had been taking Dr. —'s 'periodical drops' for two weeks and that [he] should leave her alone until she had aborted."[58] While many women probably did try to determine how their pregnancies failed and considered their work habits, illnesses, and activities, Stolz also presents another possible reason for clear causation: the need to convince others that the loss was accidental. Between the 1860s and the 1880s, every state in the nation considered the legality of what some doctors referred to as "criminal abortion," and by the end of the nineteenth century, every state had a law on the books that outlawed intentional abortion at any time during pregnancy, which may have put many miscarriages under closer scrutiny. It is possible that other women provided causes to their doctors in order to prevent any suspicion of their situation. Stolz's actions are perhaps more understandable in light of the pressure Ohio's state medical society put on the state legislature to pass an antiabortion law, which was accomplished the year after Stolz reported this case.[59]

These long lists of causes also appeared in domestic health guides advising readers on the proper lifestyle of pregnant women. While the lists themselves differed little between medical texts and popular health books (aside from, perhaps, the not surprising use of "scientific"-sounding anatomical and physiological terms), the genre of the book alters the message conveyed by the long lists. In texts such as Thomas Cock's *A Manual of Obstetrics*, these lists were presentations by older, experienced practitioners who were sharing with younger students all the possibilities (even if very slight) that could lead to an unfortunate event. The longer the list, the more authoritative and experienced the author might sound, and the better prepared the student could be for any eventuality. However, within a book such as Alfred Hall's *The Mother's Own Book and Practical Guide to Health*, these lists instead became instructions for pregnant women on how to ensure their pregnancies lasted the full nine months. In this context, surely some women viewed such long lists of causes as daunting, overwhelming, and impossible to avoid. After all, how could a pregnant woman follow the advice of obstetrician Pye Henry Chavasse who warned against "anything and everything" that could possibly affect either the mind or the body?[60]

In 1849, physician and popular author Frederick Hollick published *The Matron's Manual of Midwifery*, a guide "especially intended for the instruction of females themselves." In his section on miscarriage, Hollick briefly detailed the definition of miscarriage and the point of pregnancy in which a woman was most likely to miscarry (six months), but he then quickly launched into a six-page description of the causes. On his list, Hollick included violent bodily exertions, strong mental excitement, tumors, womb diseases, corsets and tight dressing, consumption, frightful dreams, and living in certain localities. In reference to the effects of sexual intercourse on pregnancy, he also confusingly informed his readers "in some persons miscarriage is caused by a *too eager* gratification of certain desires but in others it may arise *from the opposite cause*."[61] For his readers, this cautionary list might have seemed perplexing in the least, and possibly even spelling out certain doom—for how were you to know if you were a person affected by too much or too little gratification? What was the appropriate amount of "certain desires"?

Like the authors of medical texts, authors of domestic health guides also focused on living in excess as a danger to a pregnancy. Sexual intercourse, joy, grief, blood, nervousness, and evacuations all appeared as threats when in excess.[62] Health writers also informed women of the dangers of "violent" activities, such as violent exercise, violent emotions, violent shocks to the nervous system, violent exertion, and violent fits of passion.[63] Ideas of overexertion or overexcitement also appeared with some regularity in these works.[64] In keeping with this model of balance in health,

Dr. John C. Gunn, perhaps the best-known author of domestic health guides at the time, advised his readers that pregnancy loss could result from "an over-full habit."[65] Unfortunately, Gunn did not explain further what that could mean.

One of the more predominant themes of these lists was an emphasis on balance. Doctors portrayed a woman preparing to give birth as an unsteady body that was liable to be overset by the smallest of things, as revealed in their often-contradictory advice. Proper behavior during pregnancy depicted in these miscarriage discussions reads like the Goldilocks tale—everything must be "just right." For instance, excess of blood could cause a miscarriage, but so could anemia.[66] Overexertion in walking, running up stairs, or horseback riding were deemed dangerous, and yet so was too little exercise.[67] Work was often listed as a cause as were amusements and "luxurious habits."[68] According to doctors, pregnancy could only last the necessary nine months if a woman figured out the careful balance of every activity she carried out. Should she slip up in any way—too hot or too cold—all would be lost.

Many popular guides also warned against excessive intercourse or any sexual intercourse as a threat to this unstable body.[69] Some physicians wrote euphemistically, perhaps with a nod to their more public audience, as John Gunn did in 1862 when he advised against "too much connection with your husband."[70] Pye Henry Chavasse was not as gentle or indirect: "Sexual intercourse should . . . be carefully avoided; indeed, the patient ought to have a separate bed—this is most important advice." He continued to outline the dangers of sex and closed his advice with, perhaps for some, a preposterous, if not impossible, solution: "the best plan that she can adopt will be TO LEAVE HER HUSBAND FOR SEVERAL MONTHS."[71]

Medical advice on sexual intercourse was not limited to miscarriage prevention in the nineteenth century. Particularly in the last half of the century, health guide readers would have been able to find numerous connections between health and sexual activity.[72] In 1831, Charles Knowlton first published *Fruits of Philosophy*, his pathbreaking work that brought science to sexual relations in approachable language.[73] While the book is most often credited with providing American couples with birth control advice, it served an important role as the first work to frankly and openly discuss sex in a popular health guide.[74] Following in Knowlton's wake, various groups and writers began to advise American couples on sexual habits, sexual frequency, and fertility control.

A major aspect of these new conversations about sex was reform physiology, a movement, directed mostly at the emerging middle class, which revealed the inner workings of the human body in nonscientific language. Often, these revelations included frank discussions of sex, conception, and how to prevent pregnancy. In 1834, Sylvester Graham, the popular health reformer (and inventor of graham crackers), informed his readers that sexual desire could lead to "debility, disordered functions, and permanent disease"; his list of the possible results of marital sexual excess included general debility, indigestion, feebleness of circulation, hysterics, impaired vision, weakness of the lungs, disorders of the liver and kidneys, and weakness of the brain.[75] It is easy to see how pregnancy loss could fit within such a list. William Alcott, another popular writer of nineteenth-century health guides, agreed with Graham's depictions of the dangers of sexual excess in marriage. While his advice for sexual regularity was not as clear as that offered by Graham (who recommended married couples have sex only once a month), Alcott described numerous cases of men who were brought low by their overabundance in the marital bed.[76] Other writers and reformers connected sex and ill health in a variety of ways, and although there was sometimes disagreement among the reformers on how sex affected health and the rest of the body, all did agree that there was an important link to be made.[77]

All of this popular advice for avoiding miscarriage provides insight into what physicians believed constituted a healthy, but also a proper pregnancy. Indeed, much of this advice derived from the image of proper femininity in nineteenth-century America. Women should not show immoderate emotion (violent passions, excessive joy), physically exert themselves (running, horseback riding), or show signs of a sexual nature. Above all, the female body, especially during pregnancy, was extraordinarily fragile. Not only was this notion supported by the miscarriage cases doctors actually saw—such as where a pregnancy loss could destroy a woman's body—but also by social messages that dictated that women stay at home and be "protected" from the strains of economic and political decisions.

This image of proper femininity, however, was modeled on the urban middle class and may not have been attainable to many readers of domestic health guides who bought the books because they could not afford a physician or because they could not find one near their rural home. Many authors warned against the luxuries of the upper class. Mary Melendy warned against parties, balls, and concerts in her advice on keeping a pregnancy safe.[78] Alfred Folger cautioned against "high living," and John Gunn informed his readers of the risks of "luxurious habits."[79] Joseph Pulte was perhaps the most vocal proponent of avoiding amusements or indulgences. He claimed that "a weakening, luxurious mode of living" caused pregnancy loss, and he argued that these "artificial means of producing life's fleeting pleasures" should be discarded in favor of the "more lasting joys" of motherhood. Pulte advised his readers to "cheerfully forgo for a short time, the fashionable and doubtful amusements of so-called fashionable society" in order to protect a pregnancy, and perhaps become a socially appropriate mother.[80]

Other authors listed suspected causes that were clearly directed at upper-class women, such as "high living," dancing, riding in carriages, "luxurious habits," and sea-bathing.[81] Throughout the second half of the nineteenth century, American physicians painted a portrait of miscarriage as an evil primarily because it was a threat to a certain group of women and families, namely, the white, native-born, middle and upper class. In his 1871 guide, *A Physician's Counsels to Woman*, Walter Taylor warned his readers that mental agitation was a common cause of miscarriage, but rather than describing the dangers of agitation brought on by worry over work, food, or other mental drains of the working class, Taylor instead focused on the perils of "fictitious emotions produced by the sensational novel and drama."[82]

In the end, there are multiple reasons why these extensive lists of causes failed to convince women that physicians had expertise in understanding miscarriage. For women who did not spend their pregnancies attending balls, reading sensational novels, or pursuing any number of other amusements of fashionable society, these lists would have seemed irrelevant and thus useless. But for most women, the sheer volume of potential causes of miscarriage could have made this expert advice confusing, overwhelming, and impossible to follow. While physicians may have thought that such thorough lists could convince women that male doctors had extensive knowledge and thus surely could help them in cases of pregnancy loss, the lists instead might have convinced women that miscarriage was common and unavoidable. In the end, if miscarriage was just a routine part of being a reproducing woman in nineteenth-century America, why would you need a doctor?

Living Pregnantly

Although authors of popular health guides in the 1840s began presenting their female readers with long lists of all the behaviors, activities, and unpredictable and uncontrollable events that could alter pregnancy and steer it down a dangerous path, a glimpse into the daily lives of pregnant women uncovers little acknowledgment or adoption of such advice. The lists of pregnancy-loss causes and prevention advice provided in teaching texts and domestic health guides presented a view of the nineteenth-century pregnant woman as besieged on all sides, with threats to her pregnancy around every corner. Almost anything could upset the delicate balance of pregnancy, at least according to these mostly male medical writers. According to reproducing women, however, these threats played little role in daily life. Many women continued to live their lives unchanged once they determined they were pregnant.

Rachel Bowman Cormany provides a good example of the unanalyzed life of a pregnant woman in the nineteenth century. A university graduate, Rachel Bowman married fellow schoolmate Samuel Cormany in late 1860. While honeymooning in her home country of Canada, the Cormanys decided to remain north a bit longer as war broke out in the United States. Samuel was unable to find work, so Rachel began to seek out pupils for art lessons, even during her advancing pregnancy. As she actively worked to get more students and spent many hours a day teaching, she lamented that she was "quite unwell," and "quite sick tired & lame," but on December 2, 1862, she wrote in her diary of her success at going out and soliciting pupils. She reported: "felt so elated at my success that I think I shall start out soon again to get some more. I can teach a dozen as well as one, which would make quite a difference in the purse at the end."[83] Toward the end of her pregnancy, Cormany even found herself bartering art lessons to a relative in return for help during the birth, but she was informed that the price was still too steep. Cormany lamented in her journal, "I think it is hard to do any thing cheap enough for relatives."[84]

Alice Bodman provides another example of a woman who made few changes to her daily activities during pregnancy. Married to Joseph Bodman in 1882, Alice quickly became pregnant, giving birth to a son fifteen months after her wedding. Throughout her pregnancy, Bodman continued a myriad of household chores, including cooking, cleaning, sewing, and mending, as well as making clothing for elderly women in the community. Alongside these laborious chores, Bodman also continued working as a piano teacher throughout her pregnancy. Joseph Bodman was frequently ill, and the couple often depended on Alice's income for basic necessities. On April 7, just a few weeks before giving birth, Bodman recorded in her diary: "Busy with the regular routine of housework again today. Gave Ada Ruby her music lesson this afternoon as usual. . . . Helped Mother get the supper, and also helped to do up the supper dishes." Bodman believed so strongly that her work should go on as usual, despite what some would call her "delicate" condition, that on January 16 she wrote, "Crocheted all the morning and slept nearly all afternoon. A very lazy record. Am ashamed of it."[85]

Other women wrote of carrying out their daily tasks of sewing, cooking, cleaning, and often working long days throughout their pregnancies.[86] Some even traveled extensively, frequently exhausting themselves, but they rarely expressed fears of the result their activities may have had on their pregnancies. Elizabeth Cabot not only continued her usual household duties, but she also took an extended vacation to Europe during her third pregnancy in 1869. Visiting numerous countries, Cabot took long walks, rode in carriages and on horseback, and often stayed up until after midnight—activities that doctors frequently warned against as causes of pregnancy loss. Cabot wrote of an easy birth in Paris, soon after arriving to the city. Overall, Cabot seemed to give little consideration to her pregnancy in her travel planning.[87]

Emily McCorkle FitzGerald also found herself with extensive travel plans while pregnant in 1874.[88] Shortly after the birth of her first child, FitzGerald's husband, an army doctor, was assigned to a camp in Sitka, Alaska. When she was three months pregnant, FitzGerald boarded a ship in New York and sailed for Sitka. This journey included a three-hour trek across the Panama isthmus, as well as stops in San Francisco and Portland. FitzGerald reported some seasickness while sailing, but her greatest concern was reaching Alaska before giving birth. Once in Sitka, FitzGerald quickly became busy setting up her house, cooking, sewing, and caring for her one-year-old daughter. She also was cooped up in the house for many days while workers painted her new rooms. Although FitzGerald probably had little choice in the matter, she never mentioned the possibility of restricting any of her activities because of her pregnancy, nor did she express any worry about the effects of her strenuous schedule. She gave birth two months after arriving at her new home.

Some women did restrict their activities during pregnancy, but usually it was based on what they felt they were physically capable of, not on any notion of what was proper or safe for a pregnant woman. Toward the end of her pregnancy, Blanche Ames began to curtail one of her normal pursuits, which she reported to her husband, "Mother and the boys have gone to church, Del. Mrs. Butler was too lazy, and I too <u>stout</u>, to do duty in that direction."[89] Her husband responded, "So the 'cove' has become tiresome physically?

I am disposed to resent that and tell him he had 'better mind his own business' and not be making people wearied and tired."[90]

Ellen Wright Garrison was forced to cease some of her social activities during her pregnancy, but not out of any sense of duty or pregnancy-loss avoidance. Garrison, married to William Lloyd Garrison (son to the prominent abolitionist of the same name), was pregnant with her fifth child in 1879 when she wrote to her sister, Eliza Wright Osborne, about missing her brother-in-law's wedding: "I was too deadly sick to go! Six weeks along & can't swallow a morsel but gruel & the like! I'm very glad to! But this part of it is very distressing. It seems impossible that I can get to Ashburn, & after I get there will be still more embarrassing, for I can't go near the table, or even sit straight in a chair, but have to lie down nearly all the time!"[91] Garrison gave birth to her youngest daughter, Eleanor, eight months later. Katherine Norton disclosed the limits to a favored activity of many nineteenth-century women in a letter to her cousin: "It's terribly hard to write because the desk and I meet in the middle and the inkstand is almost out of reaching distance."[92]

Most of the women I studied made no mention of curtailing activities out of a sense of duty or fear of pregnancy failure. For a few, fatigue, illness, or size may have placed restrictions on certain undertakings, but for most, life continued as usual. The one exception to this trend was Katherine Norton, who in a letter to her cousin Agnes Garrison in 1898 wrote: "It is a real blow to think that when this reaches you, you will see Charley [Norton's husband] without me,—or rather that he will see you while I won't. . . . The cause of it all is—as perhaps you know already—the presence of a little Norton which (since it won't be 'who' until December) makes any more traveling than is absolutely necessary rather risky."[93] Norton was the only woman to speak of risk in pregnancy. None of the other women I studied expressed concern over a precarious situation, one that required protection. It should be pointed out, however, that Norton's letter is the latest of all of the personal writings, and thus it is plausible that she represents the beginning of a shift in pregnancy thinking. Perhaps more women were beginning to consider risks and to guard their pregnancies by the turn of the twentieth century.

Finally, the case of Dolly Lunt Burge presents another interpretation of the role of causation in cases of miscarriage: miscarriage was uncontrollable, at least by mere mortals, so why even ponder causation? The daughter of a local merchant, Dolly Lunt was born in Maine, where she met Samuel Lewis, who became a devoted, if not a somewhat financially irresponsible, suitor. At twenty-one Lunt finally agreed to marry Lewis, and less than a year later, their first child was born. Little Samuel lived only a few months, but in 1840 Dolly Lewis again gave birth, this time to a daughter. After difficulties finding work, Samuel Lewis moved his family south in 1842, settling in Georgia, where he embarked on a medical career. This career did not prove to be very profitable, and so Dolly Lewis began teaching at a local academy. She became pregnant again, but the new baby, born in 1843, died within hours of its birth. Only five months later, Samuel died as well, from congestive fever. The following year, Lewis lost her daughter who died of bronchitis at the age of three. By 1848, Lewis was alone in Georgia.[94]

The next time Dolly Lunt Lewis became pregnant, her life was very different. Following the loss of her family, Lewis, taking pride in being able to provide for herself, continued working in Georgia. In 1848, she met Thomas Burge, a recently widowed wealthy planter with four children, and in January 1850, they were married. At the age of thirty-three, Burge was pregnant for the fourth time, but she had no living children. After announcing her pregnancy in her diary in December 1850, Burge recounted, over the next five months, settling into her new home, her relations with her new stepchildren, and her ill health. On May 12, 1851, she wrote, "The second day of this month was taken sick & after several hours of severe pain [gave] premature birth to a daughter. True I had all along feared it would be thus but was not resigned to the dispensation. I would rather suffered three months longer if then I could have had my living daughter but God knows what is best for us."[95]

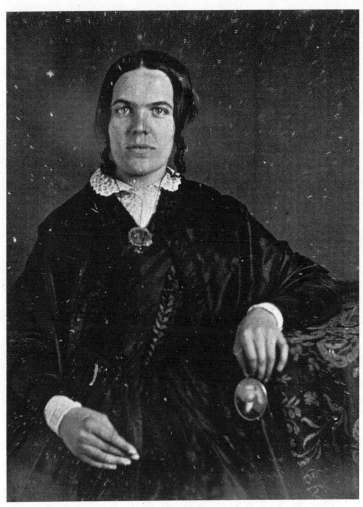

FIG. 5. Dolly Lunt Burge (undated). (Burge Family Papers, Stuart A. Rose Manuscript, Archives, and Rare Books Library, Emory University)

Burge, a devout Methodist, understood her loss as the will of God and out of her control. Rather than looking to any action during her pregnancy or a discernible cause, she interpreted the event in terms of a larger divine plan for her life. While nineteenth-century women created various meanings for their pregnancy losses, many, like Burge, kept preventability out of the picture. For some women, even for those not so inclined to look for divine intervention, the idea that miscarriage was uncontrollable was supported by the popular health literature. One way to interpret the long lists of "everything and anything" causes for miscarriage was that the pregnant body was delicate and unstable, requiring intense protection and expert guidance—probably the reading most physicians were hoping for. But for some women, another interpretation of those long lists was that because miscarriage could be caused by, as one physician argued, "almost every action of daily life," attempts to determine cause, or avoid them, were fruitless exercises.[96]

Call the Doctor

Prior to the 1830s, most domestic health guides that addressed miscarriage gave instructions for how to care for a woman who might be losing her pregnancy. By the middle of the century, however, families would have been hard pressed to find such advice. Most of the domestic health literature published between 1830 and 1870 instead provided a very simple directive in the case of miscarriage: call a doctor. In these popular books physicians clearly claimed special expertise when it came to miscarriage, reshaping the experience as a medical, not domestic, problem.

In 1807, Washington physician James Ewell published his first health guide, *Planter's and Mariner's Medical Companion*. By 1822, Ewell's book, now renamed *The Medical Companion, or Family Physician*, had become one of the most successful comprehensive family health guides in the new country and was in the sixth edition.[97] In the text, he included a five-page section on miscarriage. After a brief definition and description of the phenomenon, he presented his readers with a relatively short list of causes, among them severe exercise, fits of passion, "excessive venery," injuries, and stimulating medicines. He then followed with advice on how to treat miscarriage, recommending immediate bed rest, application of cold cloths to the belly and back, bleeding or giving laudanum depending on the cause, and "injecting three or four times a-day up the vagina a solution of alum." He continued to describe how to determine if miscarriage was inevitable, and if so, how to deliver the "ovum" and finish by plugging the vagina with cloth to stem the subsequent bleeding. At no point in his instructions did he advise the reader to seek out a doctor or other medical help; instead, he implied that miscarriage was a case that could be handled at home by family members equipped with his book.[98]

Another early health writer, John Gunn, published his first guide in 1830 and soon replaced Ewell as the medical author found in most American homes. Like Ewell, Gunn provided lengthy instructions on how to treat a miscarriage, including bleeding, keeping the bowels open, and liberal use of sweet oil rubbed on the back, loins, and belly. Gunn informed his readers "if these means fail in preventing the abortion, nature will effectuate the expulsion of the child . . . she may, however, be assisted in her exertions." He then detailed how the average family might help with nature. Again, he did not instruct the reader to call on a doctor and in fact relayed the advice of Samuel Bard, who wrote what was perhaps the first teaching text on midwifery in the United States, that is, a book meant for students of medicine, not American families.[99] Gunn not only saw no need for a medical practitioner in the case of miscarriage, but he also viewed the prevailing "medical" procedures as simple enough for families to carry out on their own.

Authors of domestic health guides in the 1840s and 1850s began to limit instructions on miscarriage treatment. In his popular 1847 book, New York physician Edward Dixon informed his readers of the numerous causes of miscarriage and then provided some treatment advice. However, unlike earlier authors, Dixon only included directions to have the patient lie down in a well-ventilated room. He indicated that there were many other means available to prevent or treat miscarriage, but because they were "exclusively medical in character," he would not enumerate them in this popular guide. Instead, Dixon focused on preparing the patient for the arrival of the physician.[100] Such warnings became customary over the next few decades, providing American families with little medical advice on how to treat miscarriage on their own, instead focusing on how serious the case could be—serious enough to require a doctor. Stephen Tracy, professor of obstetrics at the New England Female Medical College, informed his readers that at the very first symptoms of miscarriage, a pregnant woman should immediately send for a doctor; if she reached the second stage of miscarriage, she needed "prompt and vigorous practice on the part of the medical attendant," and if she still ignored the advice and reached the third stage of miscarriage, "it only remain[ed] for the medical attendant to conduct his patient safely through to the end."

While physicians took pride in reporting cases in which numerous women and families did call for their aid in the event of miscarriage, women's personal papers bring us a different story: the many families disappointed by the medical "help" they received. Six years later, and living only about one hundred miles away from Dolly Burge, fellow Georgian Gertrude Thomas had a miscarriage. Like Burge, Thomas kept a regular diary, detailing the activities of her family. In 1856, that family included her husband, her three-year-old son, Turner, and her parents, who owned a nearby plantation. Unlike Burge, Thomas had been raised in Southern gentility and had never had to work or want for anything. Her lifestyle would have more closely resembled that of Lucretia Everett than the lean years of Dolly Burge. And like Everett, Thomas called on a doctor when she began to suspect her pregnancy would not continue.

In July 1856, Thomas noted in her diary: "Again, I have prospects of becoming a mother and the idea (aside from the fear of accident and the natural shrinking from pain) causes pleasurable emotions. I do not wish an only child, yet I should not object to long intervals. I think Mr. Thomas views the subject with the same idea of myself and is gratified at the prospect. I have as yet mentioned this to no one but himself."[101] A month later, Thomas accompanied her husband, father-in-law, and brother-in-law on a trip to a nearby plantation. The trip required a two-mile ride in the carriage, an arduous one for a pregnant woman according to most physicians, but Thomas reported: "the day passed pleasantly [and] the dinner was very nice." Upon returning to her husband's parents' house, Thomas found herself so fatigued as to forgo "the party after tea in the Piazza," and she retired early for the night.

She later wrote, "early the next morning I found that I was in such a situation as to frighten me with fears of sickness. Coming up home we called by for Dr Eve. Nothing that he did (in fact he did nothing) proved efficacious, and on Monday I had an abortion—at two months." Recounting that she "was not very much frightened," but suffered "extreme debility," Thomas closed the entry with an account of her time in her sickbed: "I have had a good deal of company and Ma has been kind in supplying me with grapes, peaches and &c."[102]

While Thomas described her travels and the fatigue that immediately preceded her miscarriage, she never directly linked the activities to her lost pregnancy, and in fact she showed no interest in considering how her miscarriage originated. In a later pregnancy, Thomas grew somewhat fearful at a constant pain in her stomach, explaining, "I have been so unfortunate in having a premature birth and an abortion that being in a similar state I naturally fear a similar accident."[103] Rather than connecting her abortion to any discernible cause, Thomas instead resigned herself to being unfortunate. Like Burge, Thomas perhaps understood her lost pregnancy to be out of her control and mostly inexplicable.

Conclusion

Like Abigail Adams and Lucretia Everett, Gertrude Thomas followed the advice of so many American physicians and health writers by calling for a doctor, but she was left with no pregnancy and little confidence in the medical field. While American physicians sought to convince women and their families of the value of medicine in the case of miscarriage, these efforts largely failed. Upper-class women such as Gertrude Thomas, Lucretia Everett, and Abigail Adams continued to call for a doctor when a pregnancy came to an untimely end, but these women were following an older social convention, not acting out of a perceived necessity for medical aid. And in fact, when faced with the seemingly impotent "aid" of their physicians, these women expressed frustration, disappointment, and distrust in the skill of practitioners.

Meanwhile, lower-class women like Dolly Burge saw no reason to call on a doctor in the event of a miscarriage. Burge hoped her pregnancy would last the full nine months, and after losing her first three children, she yearned for a child, but she saw no value in medical aid and suffered through her miscarriage with only the help of her husband by her bed. Doctors in the middle of the nineteenth century had nothing effective, or even perceived to be effective, to offer women like Burge. By crafting the image of miscarriage as *always* being a dangerous condition, and by claiming they possessed special knowledge about the causes of miscarriage, doctors hoped to become the ultimate arbiters of pregnancy loss, but these arguments largely fell on deaf ears. Women like Gertrude Thomas, Abigail Adams, and Lucretia Everett wanted doctors who did something to stop their miscarriages; they looked for doctors to take action, not pontificate on whether it was a strong odor or a sudden fright that caused the incident.

In a lecture to students in 1851, the influential obstetrician Charles Meigs claimed that too many women ended up "in the hands of the quack," who lead them "by gradual lapses of health and strength, down to the grave, the last refuge of the incurable, or rather the uncured."[104] Meigs was speaking on the general category of diseases of women, but many physicians shared his sentiments, especially when it came to miscarriage. While generally unsuccessful at convincing the American public that all cases of miscarriage required expert medical attention, doctors could still rely on the pain, hemorrhaging, and infection of some cases to propel women to seek them out. It would take larger social and demographic changes to move medicine to the center of miscarriage treatment.

4

Dr. Taylor Went Up in the Uterus

Miscarriage Treatment and Intrusive
Interventions, 1860–1900

In June 1846, eighteen-year-old and newly married Susan Shelby Magoffin opened her diary and wrote excitedly: "My journal tells a story tonight different from what it has ever done before. The curtain rises now with a new scene. This book of travels is *Act 2nd*, literally and truly. From the city of New York to the Plains of Mexico, is a stride that I myself can scarcely realize."[1] Magoffin was embarking on what would become an eighteen-month trip along the Santa Fe Trail, from Missouri into Chihuahua, Mexico, with her husband, Samuel, a veteran trader and his brother, James Magoffin, a government agent hoping to smooth the way for American occupation of New Mexico. Born to a wealthy family in Kentucky, Magoffin described her excitement in leaving civilization to undertake the next chapter of her life: frontier travel with her dashing husband. Over the next six weeks, the Magoffins, setting off from Independence, Missouri, traveled across Kansas and into Colorado, where they stopped for a few weeks before turning south along the Sangre de Cristo Mountains to Santa Fe. Their stop was at Bent's Fort, an important fur-trading camp and base on the Santa Fe Trail, where they were given a spacious room, and Susan could socialize with other ladies in the parlor and discuss life on the Western frontier.

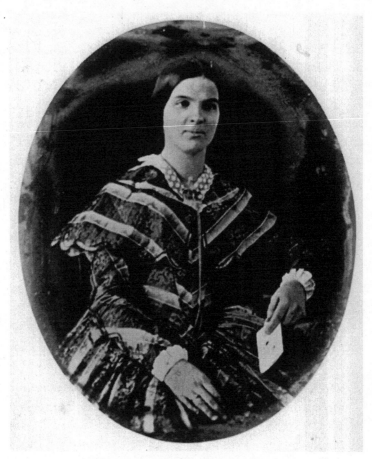

FIG. 6. Susan Shelby Magoffin (ca. 1850). (Missouri History Museum, St. Louis)

A few days after arriving at the fort, Magoffin noted a visit by the fort physician, a Dr. Mesure. Writing with a bit more levity than was common for her journal, Magoffin confessed that on setting out on this major trip, she had hoped the travel and climate would prove good for her health, which had been weak in the past few years. Unfortunately, her hopes, she wrote, had been "blasted," for she was "rather going down hill than up."[2] Two days later, on her nineteenth birthday, she revealed another aspect of her delicate health: "I feel rather strange, not at its [her birthday] coming, nor to think that I am growing rather old, for that is the way of the human family, but this is it, I am sick!"[3] Relying on a common nineteenth-century convention, Magoffin used the term "sick" to indicate that she was pregnant. Based on later entries, she was somewhere between three and five months along at the time.

The next morning, however, Magoffin awoke with sharp pains and soon understood what was happening to her body, or rather, to her pregnancy. A week later she recorded: "In a few short months I should have been a happy mother and made the heart of a father glad, but the ruling hand of a mighty Providence has interposed and by an abortion deprived us of the hope, the fond hope of mortals!"[4] Magoffin, after a day of pains, which stopped when *all was over*," remained in her bed for a week, under the supervision of Dr. Mesure. She reflected on her situation, and those of women of her class, when she became aware of the circumstances in the room below hers. "An Indian woman," Magoffin wrote, "gave birth to a fine healthy baby, about the same time, *and in half an hour after she went to the River and bathed herself and it*." Magoffin expressed her amazement at the immediate recovery of the woman below and other tales of Native women bathing in frozen ponds soon after giving birth. As her own health seemed so slow to mend, and the woman below returned to normal life so quickly, Magoffin concluded that "no doubt many ladies in civilized life are ruined by too careful treatments during child-birth," whereas for the "heathen" there seemed to be nothing disadvantageous about such "heathenish" customs.[5] Tragically, nine years later back in the "civilized" world of Missouri, Magoffin died due to complications of the birth of her fourth child.[6]

This story of an upper-class white woman who found herself sharing a reproductive experience with a Native American woman on the edges of the American frontier serves as a good representation of the medical and social changes afoot in the United States in the middle of the nineteenth century. By 1850, the United States was experiencing rapid industrialization and saw unprecedented immigration, altering the logistics and the meaning of family and reproduction. As manufacturing increased with the Industrial

Revolution (beginning in the 1830s), workers moved into cities, collected higher wages, and the "middle class" emerged as families with money to spend in new stores on the plethora of commercial goods available in cities. These families, however, were also newly separated from their extended families back on the farms, which restricted their access to traditional and folk knowledge of health, illness, and miscarriage.[7] The country's population had quadrupled since the early 1800s, and now over 15 percent of citizens lived in cities. Immigration rates, which had measured around 60,000 a year in 1800, sharply rose to almost 2 million newcomers a year by 1850.[8] At the same time, with westward expansion of the country, through trading routes such as the Santa Fe Trail and railroad construction, America now also included thousands of people "different" in appearance, including Hispanics, Native Americans, and Chinese.

These major demographic changes altered the medical landscape as well, particularly when it came to childbirth. For the growing numbers of urban working-class women who were separated from their female relatives by hundreds of miles or even by an ocean, gathering up trusted and experienced women for pregnancy advice and childbirth aid was no longer an option. Many women instead turned to dispensaries or hospitals—institutions not held in high regard by anyone who could afford to turn elsewhere. The preferred option, having a doctor come to one's home, required money, but charity hospitals were free.[9]

Doctors saw this demographic shift away from home health care and the emerging need for cheap medical care during childbirth as a great opportunity for training and experimenting. Young physicians and medical students could observe a live birth in an urban hospital and test out various techniques, such as forceps or the new inhaled anesthetics, ether and chloroform. For women at these hospitals, the experience could be uncomfortable (strange men looking up their skirts), painful (with little birthing experience, many physicians overused tools and their hands for internal exams and manipulations), or even deadly (effective but safe dosages of ether and chloroform were difficult to determine with certainty).[10]

The influence of male physicians on reproduction was deeply influenced by race as well as class. While physicians delivered almost 40 percent of infants in the United States by 1850, most of those cases proved to be from the very wealthy, who sought out doctors as a status symbol, or from the very poor, who could not afford the alternatives.[11] University-educated physicians, who were almost exclusively white and upper class and happily attending to patients of the same groups, suddenly encountered the reproductive needs of women of color, immigrants, and working-class families.

With the changing face of American cities, many of these white doctors, and white elites like Susan Magoffin, came into close contact with these "lesser valued" populations, creating racialized narratives and realities about miscarriage. These demographic changes increased the number of women who appealed to doctors in cases of miscarriage, but in the early years, these women remained primarily poor and/or immigrant. Women who were miles or oceans away from their families, communities, or familiar customs, looked to male physicians for action in cases of miscarriage. It is very possible that Susan Magoffin would have relied on family and friends for aid in her miscarriage had she remained in Kentucky, but at Fort Bent her only option was Dr. Mesure.

While Magoffin wrote many times of the exotic customs of the indigenous peoples she met on the Santa Fe Trail, her remarks about the native woman easily giving birth and immediately bathing in a river reflect the attitudes of many Americans of the time. Indeed, most elite physicians viewed Native Americans, as well as other groups of less social value, as hardier, able to reproduce easily, and unaffected by the bodily trials of miscarriage and childbirth.[12] In the auspicious pages of the *American Journal of Obstetrics and Diseases of Women and Children*, St. Louis physician George Engelmann presented a common argument about the reproductive woes, or lack thereof, of "primitive people," stating that most "primitive" peoples' "labor may be characterized as short and easy, accompanied by few accidents and followed by little or no prostration." Laying out the customs and traditions of many groups, from the Modoc tribe to the "savage people" of the Antilles, Engelmann argued that these groups naturally had an easier experience with pregnancy and birth. Indeed, he claimed: "the nearer civilization is approached, the more trying does the ordeal of childbirth become." Undoubtedly, Engelmann considered men and women of his own race and class as the epitome of such "civilization."[13]

This view of the hardened bodies of the "primitive" peoples that doctors encountered in miscarriage cases allowed them to intrude upon the female body in ways that would not have been as appropriate or even allowed in the case of upper-class white women. If a physician believed that the woman miscarrying in front of him was less delicate, in physical health and in sensibilities, than his private-practice patients, then he may not have thought twice about sticking one or both of his hands up into her vagina and uterus. In addition, jabbing a sharp metal instrument into her birth canal would maybe not have seemed so controversial. In contrast, when physicians attended an upper- or middle-class woman for miscarriage and birth, this encounter typically occurred in the woman's home, where she had authority and control over the experience. It is quite plausible that physicians did not consider the use of intrusive treatments in their private practices because they assumed their patients would refuse such intimate and painful procedures.

American physicians had the opportunity to see more miscarriage cases starting in the middle of the nineteenth century, and because many of those cases were women of lower classes or immigrants, doctors might have had a greater freedom to adopt miscarriage treatment protocols that middle- and upper-class patients would have been able to refuse. For the next several decades, physicians sought access to more and more miscarriage cases to increase their business, to strengthen their profession, and to acquire scientific specimens (which will be discussed in the following chapter), but this entry was greatly facilitated by the working-class and immigrant women who showed up in their offices, hospitals, and dispensaries, seeking help that they could get nowhere else. Miscarriage stories therefore can show us the important role these "devalued" women had in the process of reformulating pregnancy loss in abnormal and medical terms.

Trusting Nature

On January 2, 1852, Virginia physician P. Claiborne Gooch attended a thirty-year-old mother of three who had been "ailing and sore through the night." Although she had continued her work the following day, even while suffering fatigue and dull pain in her lower body, she did not call on Gooch until the pains became "grinding and benumbing," similar to labor pains. Gooch examined the woman and discovered her to be five to six months pregnant and passing a good deal of blood. Upon finding her cervix dilated, he determined a miscarriage would be unavoidable. In his report of this case in the *Ohio Medical and Surgical Journal* two months later, he wrote that upon this determination "I quietly took my bed-side seat till nature accomplished her duty—mine being merely to send the husband out of the room, and to inform the women that the accident must take place." He continued to watch his patient, and later that night attempted to gently remove the mass once it had descended into her vagina, but when he found that such an action was impossible without a risk of violence, he "desisted, and waited till 10 o'clock on Nature." Instead he gave her a solution of ergot, a fungus believed to induce and strengthen uterine contractions. Around midnight, the woman finally expelled the fetus, with little active aid from the doctor.[14]

G. S. Palmer described a similar case in the pages of the *Boston Medical and Surgical Journal*, and like Gooch, imparted a lesson to his professional colleagues on the ultimate success of a passive course of treatment. In April 1856, Palmer was called in to attend a woman who had been experiencing pain and discharge, along with "a strange sensation in the vagina," for the past four weeks. Palmer examined his patient and found a five-month fetus in the woman's birth canal, which he easily removed. His attempts to remove the placenta, or rather produce its expulsion with ergot, proved unsuccessful. Palmer described that "a frightful haemorrhage [*sic*] now ensued," which he treated with a tampon, but otherwise left the patient to nature, with a nurse attending her. Four days later, the nurse reported to Palmer that the patient had delivered the placenta and seemed much relieved. Palmer described this interaction with little relief himself as the placenta "had been accidentally thrown aside, although contrary to the strictest orders." Palmer was suspicious of the nurse's assertions that the entire placenta had emerged, knowing "how easily she [the nurse] might be deceived" by the tissues, but given that the hemorrhaging was subsiding, and the patient seemed to be improving, Palmer decided to agree with the nurse and determine the case closed. Four months later, however, Palmer's suspicions proved accurate when he was called in again to find the woman "flooding copiously" and finally delivering a "roundish substance" that Palmer determined to be a piece of placenta.[15]

Perhaps Palmer shared this case with other physicians primarily because it seemed to clearly prove the superiority of male physicians over that of female practitioners, like the nurse described. Palmer was able to show that through his specialized training, he could determine the true nature of what emerged from his patient's body and thus could accurately predict the case. But this case also gave him an opportunity to remind his professional readers of the power and wisdom of nature. He closed the article with the statement: "thus did nature hermetically seal up, and perfectly protect from decomposition, in a high temperature for four months, a foreign substance, which it could not throw off at the proper time; and when the system returned to a proper state and condition, she relieved herself by expelling the same."[16] Nature was smart enough to induce miscarriage when needed and even smart enough to protect a woman from possible dangerous side effects of that miscarriage (infection-causing decomposition).

In the first two-thirds of the nineteenth century, physicians typically described miscarriage as something nature was controlling, and the job of medicine was merely to assist nature. They also frequently warned of the possible dangers if the physician or midwife interfered in the process—such artificial intervention would only harm the patient. In his 1855 text, John King asserted that "all that the physician can do is to patiently await the efforts of nature, and carefully watch the hemorrhage; as a general rule, any artificial interference is highly improper."[17] Edward Rigby warned against being in a hurry "to bring away the ovum," while Alva Curtis instructed that "the exclusion of the foetus and the placenta should very generally be trusted to nature."[18] Many physicians also warned of the dangers of interfering with what was a natural process; for example, John Pearson decried "the practice of using violent and painful means, indiscriminately, for the delivery is reprehensible and should be discontinued."[19] Some doctors directly informed medical students that it was best to wait for nature in cases of inevitable miscarriage, while others described cases that exhibited this lesson. In 1868, J. T. Young presented a case in which he employed only ice and pressure for seven days until his patient finally delivered the fetus.[20] L. G. Harley went a bit further, using only gentle friction for twenty-seven days before his patient passed a placenta.[21] Prior to the 1870s, physicians seemed in agreement that miscarriage was a natural process that might require their aid, but not any aggressive action against nature.

Women Seeking Out Doctors

While American physicians in the early and mid-nineteenth century agreed that miscarriage was a natural occurrence, a method for nature to fix pregnancies that were going wrong, part of that supposition surely resulted from the small number of miscarriage cases physicians actually saw. In my survey of over 250 medical articles reporting on miscarriage from 1800 to 1912, I noted that the appearance of such cases dramatically increased after 1870. Before then, physicians were less likely to see a miscarrying woman or to be called in to help her. Reproduction throughout most of the nineteenth century in the United States was primarily a domestic practice. Women learned how to get pregnant, or how to prevent pregnancy, from their female relatives or others in women's networks in their communities, and they primarily relied on these same women for help during pregnancy, childbirth, and childcare. The last three decades of the nineteenth century, however, saw dramatic social and economic shifts that changed these domestic reproductive practices.

Massive immigration along with industrialization encouraged the movement of many young people to urban areas, especially along the East Coast of the United States. Dislocated from their families and communities, these migrants needed aid from new people and places in times of ill health or childbirth. Women who could not afford a physician or midwife, did not have the space to give birth in their homes, were separated from the assistance of family, or who could not admit their pregnancies to their family (because they were unmarried) needed a new location in which to give birth. Thus the modern maternity hospital was born. Many of these urban poor women found help in charity hospitals where they received medical assistance in return for the experience they provided to medical students and young practitioners.[22] This new location for birth also created a new power dynamic. Women and families who invited male practitioners into their homes usually retained much of the power over what that practitioner might do. If a woman did not want anesthesia or instruments used during delivery, she could more easily exert her will. In a charity hospital, where women were at the mercy of physicians, that right of refusal was much more complicated.

The rise in maternity hospitals coincided with another shift in American medicine of the late nineteenth-century: the introduction of female physicians. Elizabeth Blackwell, often credited as the first female physician in the United States, received her medical degree in 1849, and over the next few decades hundreds of women followed in her footsteps. In 1880, there were roughly 2,000 female physicians, and by 1900 that number had risen to 7,000.[23] Some of these new practitioners, like Elizabeth Blackwell and her sister Emily, established hospitals for women and children. These institutions were meant to provide care for the emerging class of women who had few resources at home for childbirth, but they were also intended to provide a space for female medical students and physicians in which to train. Slowly, coeducational institutions and women's colleges began to offer medical education for women, but most graduates in the nineteenth century faced fierce opposition to gaining clinical experience in hospitals, which saw no advantage in accepting women doctors. To combat this, physicians such as the Blackwells opened their own hospitals.

One of the Blackwells' colleagues and a prominent medical reformer in her own right, Maria Zakrzewska, opened another such institution. In 1859, Zakrzewska began teaching at the New England Female Medical College, but she left three years later, frustrated with the lack of clinical training. To help combat this problem, she established the New England Hospital for Women and Children, which opened its doors on July 1, 1862. Zakrzewska established the hospital to serve three purposes: to provide women with medical aid from female physicians; to provide educated women with an opportunity to study medicine; and to train nurses.[24] Zakrzewska described the enterprise thus: "Our hospital affords to those women especially needing the care and advice of their own sex, during sickness and in childbirth, the comforts of a home and faithful attendance at a moderate price; offering invaluable privileges to the suffering poor."[25] The hospital founders also viewed their mission as addressing some of the holes left in family care by the rapid movement of young people into the cities in search of industrial work: "This is ... the only place where a woman—not a pauper, but of narrow means—can receive the comfort and care so necessary at the period of childbirth, if she is not so fortunate as to possess a good home and friends."[26] This group also included the masses of foreign immigrants arriving in Boston in the 1860s. In 1864, the total patient population of the hospital was 2,224, with only 1,040 of those being American-born women; 685 were from Ireland, 318 were from Germany, and the rest came from a variety of countries in Western Europe and Canada.[27]

Above all, Dr. Zakrzewska sought to change ideology, to convince regular physicians and the paying public that women could be good doctors. While major acceptance of female physicians would take another century, Zakrzewska worked to create an important space for female physicians, and a space that would be deemed good enough even for male physicians.[28] She believed that with proper training, a modern scientific hospital, and economic support, female physicians could be just as successful as their male counterparts, and she set out to prove just that. In the end, she did succeed in one respect. The New England Hospital (NEH) continually had lower-than-average rates of puerperal fever than comparable maternity hospitals in Boston and elsewhere in the nation. Puerperal, or childbed fever, which had been a scourge of maternity hospitals in the United States and Europe for at least since the previous century, caused fevers, infection, and often death. In 1844, Ignaz Semmelweis, a Hungarian Jewish obstetrician teaching in a general hospital in Vienna, theorized that childbed fever was the result of some putrefaction his medical students picked up during autopsies and brought to the bed of birthing women. He instituted severe antiseptic measures in his ward (frequent hand washing with a chlorinated lime solution) and saw puerperal fever mortality rates plummet.[29] Many Western physicians, however, resisted the idea that they were the cause of such death and destruction, and so it took decades before hand washing became a routine part of attending a birth. Thus when the NEH followed Semmelweis's model thirty years later, they were still in the vanguard.

The New England Hospital was one of many institutions built in the middle of the nineteenth century that were known as voluntary hospitals. These institutions, supported by private philanthropy, ministered to a paying clientele (although, as Zakrzewska claimed, "at a moderate price") and to the industrious and worthy poor. Patrons of the hospital could endow beds either for specific workers in the households of the wealthy, or more generally for "worthy" recipients. Like many other voluntary hospitals, the NEH attempted to include moral reform in their treatment of poor, and often unwed, mothers. Part of the mission of voluntary hospitals was to uplift the poor by helping them avoid the stigmatization and trap of pauperism that came with seeking medical aid in an almshouse hospital.[30] In one respect, the NEH stood out among the increasing number of voluntary hospitals across the country in its admittance of unmarried women into its maternity ward. Zakrzewska found herself continually defending her position that single pregnant women were a part of the category of the "worthy" poor, while most other hospitals refused to admit unmarried women in labor.[31]

Maternity hospitals, including the NEH, also became a refuge for women experiencing miscarriage. On October 4, 1873, a police officer brought a seventeen-year-old single woman to the NEH. The woman was pregnant, and her clothing was soaked with blood. The hospital staff immediately put her in bed, provided her with ergot, and examined her. The woman reported that she had passed a blood clot hours before coming to the hospital, but her bleeding had continued unabated. Three hours after her entrance, the records state that the membranes hung one inch from the cervix, but no attempt was made to further extract them, and instead doctors gave her more ergot. Two days later, the membranes had descended into her lower vagina, from which doctors finally removed them. For the next few weeks, doctors continued giving the patient ergot, hot cloths on her vulva, and enemas to help regulate her bowels. The woman was finally released on October 29, twenty-five days after her admittance, and the records read, "discharged well."[32]

In the early years of the NEH maternity ward, this entry was typical for pregnancy-loss cases. Ergot proved to be the most popular treatment for bleeding, great care was paid to the regularity of the bowels, and for women further along in pregnancy, belladonna applications were given to help soothe the breasts. As in cases reported in medical journals, doctors at the NEH followed the lead of nature and rarely interfered with the natural process of miscarriage. In 1874, a thirty-three-year-old domestic worker came to the NEH in the sixth month of pregnancy, and like most miscarriage cases in the 1870s, doctors attended to her primarily with oral medications (ergot and castor oil) or topical ointments on her breasts and abdomen. The record makes no mention of any internal treatment for her miscarriage.[33]

In the NEH, as in other charity and maternity hospitals, doctors held much of the power in the clinical encounter. Patients, like the bleeding seventeen-year-old single woman, came to the NEH in desperation, seeking help that they could not get anywhere else. Such women were perhaps more likely to put up with treatments that may have seemed intrusive, uncomfortable, or even painful. Unlike upper-class women who invited doctors into their home and paid them based on satisfactory service, women entering the rooms of the NEH had little power to refuse procedures or therapies. This new clinical situation may have encouraged physicians to try a more active, intrusive approach to miscarriage.

Indeed, by the late 1880s, NEH physicians began to treat miscarriage with quick, decisive, and invasive action. In March 1889, an unmarried twenty-two-year-old domestic worker came to NEH with pains and hemorrhage. The patient reported that she had been bleeding for three days and was in her fifth month of pregnancy. With little progression in labor and no cessation of the bleeding as the evening passed, resident physician Dr. Helen Bissell "hooked her finger in the os, and drew the cervix forward and downward." This caused rapid dilation of the cervix and in less than three hours, the head of the child could be seen in the vagina. Again, the doctor used her fingers to hook onto the child and try to pull it out, but the cervix "grasped the upper half of the head." Finally, with assistance, the fetus, dead and weighing only one-half of a pound, was born. Doctors provided the woman with ergot and a warm douche to help stop the bleeding and discharged her twenty days later.[34]

This intrusion into the patient's body to accelerate the process of delivery was just the beginning of NEH doctors' adoption of what the medical literature soon dubbed the "active treatment" for pregnancy loss. Miscarriage cases typically began to involve some sort of intervention by doctors, either in extracting the fetus or cleaning out the uterus.[35] Some cases required extensive interventions. In May 1895, a married forty-three-year-old housewife in her seventh month of pregnancy came to the NEH because she had been suffering from convulsions. When her membranes ruptured that afternoon, physicians began intervening. Dr. Stella

Taylor administered chloroform while Dr. Emma Call proceeded to manually dilate her cervix. After much effort, they accomplished dilation, and then Dr. McClamont came in and administered ether for the delivery. With external manipulations by Dr. Taylor, Dr. Call was able to deliver the right foot, but found the head held tight by the cervix. Finally, the dead infant was born after almost three hours of constant active interventions by multiple physicians. The woman went home seventeen days later.[36] In another case, after a prodigious use of iodoform packing to help stem bleeding, a miscarrying woman's cervix was dilated enough so that "Dr. Taylor went up in the uterus, ruptured membranes, and brought down left foot."[37] This description, which evokes an image of a physician crawling into a uterus, while not literal, provides an apt metaphor. By the end of the nineteenth century, obstetricians and other practitioners viewed the uterus as a new land to explore. Thus whereas earlier in the century, practitioners primarily understood the uterus by external cues and expulsions provided by nature, toward the turn of the twentieth century, doctors entered the organ and experienced it directly with their own hands.[38]

In 1872, the NEH moved out of the urban center of Boston and into the suburbs of Roxbury, where it would have a larger building (with a separate maternity building), as well as a location that would attract a better clientele.[39] As a result of this move, by 1900 many more of the NEH's patients were married, native-born, and able to pay handsomely for their medical care. But this did not mean that the original targets of the NEH stopped coming in for aid. The miscarriage cases from 1870 to 1900 showed that working, unmarried, and immigrant women continued to appeal to NEH physicians for help, and this group of women living in Boston—without families nearby, without financial resources, and perhaps without any social support—became the primary source of bodies that physicians and medical students training at the NEH would use to better understand the process of miscarriage, and to determine the most effective methods of treatment.

To be sure, this shift to active treatment of miscarriage, as opposed to the passive approach of waiting on nature, developed in part as a result of the class of women who sought help at the NEH. Many of the women who arrived at the NEH in need of aid for miscarriage matched the type of patient Maria Zakrzewska had imagined: working, immigrant, young, even unmarried. For example, in February 1884, a twenty-two-year-old woman who worked making rubber coats came to the hospital. She reported that she was unmarried but pregnant and had been experiencing labor pains for the past sixteen hours. Soon after her admission, she delivered what doctors determined to be a five-month-old fetus, a girl, who had been dead for several weeks. Doctors provided the patient with potassium bromide (as a sedative), morphine, belladonna, and bandages and discharged her after eighteen days.[40] This young woman, because of either geographical distance or personal shame, was most likely separated from her family and thus relied on the NEH to act in its stead by providing basic nursing care in a time of pain and loss.

NEH physicians also attended to a twenty-two-year-old unmarried woman, helping her through a miscarriage at seven months and then treating her lacerated cervix; they admitted a twenty-two-year-old British actress who delivered a boy weighing 2¾ pounds whom they attempted to keep alive using warm water, electricity, and manual insufflation, all to no avail; and they administered to an unmarried woman working in domestic service whose bleeding required physicians to intervene with fingers and ergot and who finally delivered a five-month fetus "with well-formed fingernails."[41] These women had little social, economic, or political power in these clinical encounters, and thus physicians may have felt they had more leeway to stick their hands and instruments into their patients' bodies.

This is not, however, a story of evil doctors experimenting on powerless patients. Women, in fact, played important roles in this shift in miscarriage treatment. If a woman found herself bleeding or in pain during her pregnancy, traveled to the NEH for help and ended up merely being put in bed and given some ergot, she might have expressed dissatisfaction with the lack of medical action. I do not think Lucretia Everett was alone in her disappointment in the early passive nature of doctors in miscarriage cases. Surely some of the female patients at the NEH expected physicians to actually *do* something to help protect their pregnancies or their own health. Miscarrying women undoubtedly influenced the medical acts of physicians at the NEH, contributing to the shift in treatment that compelled doctors to "go up in" the uterus. It is also quite possible that NEH patients were more willing to allow the female NEH doctors to intrude in their bodies in such an intimate manner. Male obstetricians in the nineteenth century frequently complained of the discomfort of both patient and practitioner when they carried out vaginal examinations. Most likely, some of the female patients at the NEH felt much more comfortable having a female physician put her fingers, hands, or instruments into their uteruses than they would have with a male physician.

Not all cases required invasive action, and many medical discussions of the time centered around being able to determine the difference between inevitable and threatened miscarriage (although for the most part, the topic of threatened miscarriage appeared far less frequently in teaching texts). NEH physicians, while perhaps recognizing that the tide of modern medicine was moving toward action, still relied on passive watching when they determined it would be beneficial to their patient and her pregnancy. After four pregnancies that all resulted in miscarriage, a twenty-seven-year-old Swedish housewife sought out the medical advice of a Dr. Whitney when she experienced pain in her fourth month of pregnancy in October 1889. Dr. Whitney, recognizing "threatened abortion," brought the woman to the NEH for treatment. Over the next fourteen days, doctors kept the woman in bed, in a quiet room, and provided a liquid diet. After six days of no pain or discharge, they released her, still pregnant.[42]

Increased interactions between educated physicians and less-powerful women over miscarriage was not a trend restricted to Boston, or even to large urban centers. Many families outside of the big cities looked to physicians for aid in cases of miscarriage, such as the patients of Charles Brayton. Born to a well-to-do builder on the coast of Connecticut, Brayton decided against following his father into the masonry business and instead attended the College of Physicians and Surgeons in New York City before returning home to Stonington in 1873 to open his practice.[43] In March of that year, Brayton began to track the births he attended in a log that he kept religiously until his death in 1912 at the age of sixty-one. Along with the typical twenty to forty births that Brayton attended each year, he recorded cases of miscarriage. One of the first was the case of November 3, 1874, when Brayton visited Mary Duffy, an unmarried twenty-one-year-old woman originally from Liverpool, England. Brayton recorded "illegitimate child, mother would not tell the name of father. She had laced her corsets up at about the 3rd month and had never taken them off." Brayton delivered the premature child who he believed had been dead for at least three weeks.[44] While the total number of miscarriage cases Charles Brayton listed in his log usually comprised between only 5 and 12 percent of the total births he attended (with some years seeing no miscarriages, and three years the proportion being 18–27 percent), investigation into the cases reveals a pattern very similar to the patient population treated at the NEH.

In the last three decades of the nineteenth century, Stonington, located on the southern coast of Connecticut about sixty miles east of New Haven, served as home to many immigrants and their children who worked in the wool and cotton mills, in the vibrant shipping industry, or as servants in the houses of the upper class. In 1880, 17 percent of Stonington's 7,364 residents were foreign born, and 38 percent had at least one foreign-born parent. The town was primarily white, with only 227 residents (or approximately 3 percent of the town's residents) identified as "black" or "mulatto."[45] By comparison, of the women and families who sought out Dr. Brayton (one of nine physicians in the town) in cases of miscarriage, 47 percent were immigrants and 8 percent "colored."[46]

While working-class immigrants comprised a minority of Stonington's overall population, they ended up accounting for the majority of Brayton's patient base in cases of miscarriage. Couples such as Louis and Louise Rassum from Germany, Joseph and Delphina Maraya from the Azores, Olaf and Josephine Rood from Norway, and Michael and Catherine Harrington from Ireland all sought out Brayton for aid, most likely because they had left family and traditional healers behind in their home countries.[47] As more and more immigrant groups arrived on the shores of America, in cities like Boston but also in towns like Stonington, Connecticut, physicians' patient bases expanded dramatically. More women sought out physicians for help with miscarriage, and in turn physicians began to look at miscarriage with new eyes. Although pregnancy loss was previously understood as nature's fix to a pregnancy going bad, by the 1880s American doctors began to argue that any instance of pregnancy loss was dangerous, abnormal, and required the skilled hands and instruments of male elites. In the end, they succeeded in part not because their arguments were necessarily persuasive, but because women like Delphina Maraya had nowhere else to turn when she began bleeding in the fourth month of her pregnancy.

The Modern Miscarriage

Once American physicians began treating the growing numbers of miscarriage cases, they responded with increasingly aggressive and intrusive procedures. Only a few decades after Dr. Gooch recounted marking time patiently at the bedside of a miscarrying woman, and countless others advocated waiting for nature to take its course, the medical journals filled with stories of women treated for miscarriage with quick and invasive action. By the 1880s, probably because of patient interest and the medical views of poor, immigrant, and female patients of color, physicians began describing miscarriage as an unnatural outcome of pregnancy, a problem that only trained medical practitioners could fix. At the same time, this reshaping of miscarriage into a medical case also allowed physicians to understand miscarriage as a phenomenon of a uterus, not as an experience of a woman.

The writings of William T. Lusk serve as an example of this new approach to miscarriage. After serving in the Union army during the Civil War, Lusk pursued his medical degree at the newly founded Bellevue Hospital Medical College in New York

City (which later merged with the medical school of New York University). In 1871, he began working as professor of obstetrics and gynecology at Bellevue, where he remained on staff until his death in 1897.[48] In the 1870s, in the midst of the changing profile of miscarriage, Lusk was a practicing physician, professor of obstetrics and gynecology at a prominent East Coast hospital, and well respected, especially after the publication (and republication in many languages) of his *Science and Art of Midwifery*, a book hailed by at least one journal as "the best treatise on the subject that had ever been published."[49]

Over the course of three issues of the popular medical journal *Medical and Surgical Reporter* in December 1875, Lusk provided his instructions for determining and treating miscarriage. These three articles were based on Lusk's lectures, presumably given to medical students at Bellevue.[50] While one obituary of Dr. Lusk described him as conservative and "timid in his proving of new remedies and surgical procedures," in his lectures on miscarriage Lusk clearly supported the newer active treatment.[51] After a general discussion of the definition of miscarriage, its possible causes, and how to determine if one was occurring, Lusk detailed the frequency of the event (one in ten pregnancies) and why medical aid should always be involved: "as far as the mother is concerned, an abortion is never a matter of indifference, because of the dangers." Lusk spent the rest of his lecture (just over half of the lecture's total of thirteen pages) addressing the proper treatment. Overall, Lusk was in favor of quick and judicious intervention by a physician in cases of miscarriage, and he championed the use of the finger to remove a retained ovum or placental tissue. He also gave detailed instructions on how to properly tampon the vagina (insert damp cotton around the cervix to draw out retained tissues), dilate the vagina with a speculum, and use ergot to incite contractions as well as anesthesia to relax the abdominal muscles. He ended his advice by discussing the benefits and detriments of using ovum forceps instead of fingers, reminding his audience that later in pregnancy (after the fourth month), a practitioner could use more than one finger, and could potentially insert an entire hand into the uterus to help clean it out.[52]

These three articles reflect the transformation of the physician from acting as a helper of nature in cases of miscarriage to a man of action, fixing nature's mistake. But according to Lusk, preserving the health and even life of the patient was not the only reason to act quickly. Lusk did not leave his students wondering about the larger utility of being able to treat miscarriage cases, but he closed his speech by clearly explaining how they would benefit from this knowledge. Bringing a woman back from the seeming brink of death with the simple procedure of removing a retained ovum or placenta, Lusk informed his students, would "add more to [one's] reputation than almost any other class of cases."[53] This final statement provides further insight into much of Lusk's insistence on clearing out the uterus quickly and decisively; successfully treating miscarriage could propel the careers of his students and elevate the profession as a whole.

Lusk's lectures allow us to better appreciate how this transition from doctor as a patient helper of nature to doctor as a controlling and active agent in fixing nature also dramatically altered the understanding of the role of the female body in miscarriage. One of the more striking aspects of Lusk's writings is the relative lack of female patients. In the first article, while describing the causes and mechanisms of miscarriage, Lusk stated "here we have a uterus cut open, to expose the decidua," indicating that in his lectures, Lusk materialized miscarriage through a uterine specimen, which was detached from a woman and in fact completely devoid of any connection to a human body.[54] Throughout the rest of his lecture, as he instructed his students about rigid uterine walls, hemorrhaging, or disease, they could gaze upon this disembodied uterus as the embodiment of the entire process.

Throughout the other articles, Lusk continued to separate the uterus from any female patient, indicating to his students that they would not be treating a woman in cases of miscarriage, but instead they would be working with specified organs along with, of course, the ovum held within. When providing instructions on proper tamponing, Lusk advised his students to use whatever material may be at hand, relating that a colleague "once snatched an apron from one of the nurses and crowded it into the vagina," without any regard for how the woman in question may have felt about this action.[55] Lusk's instructions were almost solely focused on the uterus, cervix, vagina, ovum, and placenta without any reference to the comfort, relief, or response of the woman involved in all of this intervention. Even when instructing his students about anesthesia, rather than discussing how it could ease the patient, Lusk stated "anaesthesia relaxes the abdominal muscles, and enables us, with ease, to crowd down the uterus, so that the cervix is brought very near the vulva."[56]

This dehumanized discussion of uterus, cervix, and abdominal muscles surely enabled doctors to more easily adopt internal intervention in cases of miscarriage. If medical students, like those at Bellevue, learned to think of miscarriage as something that happened to an organ, and not to a woman, then it would have been easier for those practitioners to imagine sticking a metal instrument into a delicate, supremely private opening in a woman's body. Instead of seeing this version of miscarriage treatment as what could be considered the uncomfortable, perhaps even crippling, notion of not only looking under a woman's skirt, but also putting one's hands into her vagina, Lusk's treatment crafted the practice as a manipulation of a body part that could not shrink back in shame, make any noise in surprise, fear, or pain, and that could not express any negative response to the physician's actions.

Lusk was not alone in teaching or practicing this new intrusive treatment on disembodied organs. By the 1870s, doctors began to argue that they needed to take a more active role and relegate nature and their patients largely to the background. While in the 1850s and 1860s it was routine for physicians to wait upon, or aid, nature, by the end of the nineteenth century medical writings show a marked trend toward supporting actively intervening and emptying the uterus.[57] At an 1879 meeting of the Norfolk Medical Society, Henry Martin claimed that in all cases of pregnancy loss, "the one thing essential in the treatment ... [is] to empty the uterus as soon as that can be done with safety, to thoroughly ascertain that it is entirely emptied and never to cease supervision of the case until that end is accomplished." In his presentation, Martin described women whose lives were in danger because of physicians who followed a more passive practice, who did not enter the woman's body and pull out all that they could, or who disdained tools like forceps. It is important to note, however, that Martin also believed that "honest miscarriage" (as opposed to "dishonest" or induced abortion) was very frequent "among the lower laboring classes."[58] Thus the bodies Martin worked with, or envisioned entering with forceps and fingers, were the bodies of women who had little social power. Martin was not advocating that such quick and intrusive action be taken among women who invited him into their homes and paid him handsomely. The increased interaction between male physicians and poor miscarrying women enabled the growing popularity of intrusive action to treat miscarriage.

In 1897, Henry Garrigues also strongly advocated an active treatment to miscarriage, claiming: "the sooner the uterus is emptied the better it will be for the patient." Garrigues informed the readers of *Medical News* that in most of the miscarriage cases he saw, he dilated the cervix manually (using a series of hard rubber dilators) and emptied the uterus, using a large dull wire curette. Curettes were long, thin, metal instruments, often with a curved end, that could be used to scrape along the uterine wall. Using words like "violence," "scraping," and "force," Garrigues builds a portrait of miscarriage treatment that would probably have seemed uncomfortable to most patients, even unbelievable to many. But Garrigues was the consulting obstetric surgeon to a New York maternity hospital. Most of the miscarrying women he encountered in his practice probably had little say in the treatment they received, and Garrigues may have assumed their lower-class bodies were hardy enough to accept the violence and force of his treatments that scraped the inside of their uteruses with a dull curette.[59]

At the same time, this new interest in intrusive treatment was also enabled by where physicians encountered miscarriage. In his

1863 teaching manual, New York obstetrician Gunning S. Bedford proposed a question to his students: "imagine you are at the bedside of a pregnant female, who has both pain and a discharge of blood from the vagina, and that you have satisfactorily ascertained, through a carefully instituted examination, that these two phenomena are positively connected with a threatened miscarriage—what is the first thing to be done?" He answered this question by recommending the physician conduct a careful survey of the patient, taking into consideration her temperament, her recent lifestyle, her emotional state, and her medical history. Certainly, Bedford was not endorsing quick and decisive action, and indeed he cautioned his students: "[do] not, for the mere sake of appearing to do something, be urged on to precipitate and unprofitable interference." But we need to take note of the image he painted for his students: that of a practitioner at a woman's bedside. By the 1880s, more and more physicians were facing miscarriage cases not at a woman's bedside but in a maternity hospital or dispensary. This change of location meant that physicians no longer had the leisure nor the motivation to indulge in a lengthy survey of a patient's life; instead, they could quickly move to insert sharp metal instruments into her vagina. In addition, many of these new patients were poor, immigrant, and generally of "lower stock" than many upper-class white physicians imagined themselves to be.

To be sure, some of the rise in this direct intervention was a reaction to the cases doctors encountered. As early as the 1850s, American doctors detailed in the pages of medical journals cases wherein women's lives were endangered by miscarriage. In 1865, Dr. Thaddeus Leavitt, attending physician to the Germantown Dispensary in Philadelphia, visited Mrs. A., who was in her sixth month of pregnancy. Mrs. A. had called for medical aid after vomiting, suffering abdominal pains, and experiencing "great prostration" for two weeks. Leavitt initially gave the patient opium and mustard applications—common nonintrusive therapies. Mrs. A. seemed relieved by these efforts, but she called for the doctor again four days later when she was "in a state of collapse" after delivering the "contents of the uterus." Mrs. A. remained in a critical state for many days after, but she eventually made a thorough recovery. Dr. Leavitt was pleased to report of her eventual good health, proved by another pregnancy nine months later.[60] While Leavitt followed a more conservative, nonintrusive plan of treatment, he perhaps noticed that the woman's affliction was finally abated only after she delivered fetal and placental tissues. After weeks of illness, Mrs. A.'s health, and possibly even life, was saved by emptying her uterus.

In the next few decades doctors altered their response to miscarriage, advocating a more active plan of attack, and they could often show the benefit of such a plan. Many physicians encountered cases involving dangerous symptoms from miscarriage, and their reliance on speed and action certainly helped save many lives. In 1889, a messenger awoke Dr. C. H. Shivers and requested his presence at the home of a Mrs. P., who, the messenger reported, "was bleeding to death." Mrs. P. had miscarried at two and half months almost two months prior and had seemingly recovered easily until the recent bleeding. Shivers found Mrs. P. "nearly bled out" and quickly diagnosed retained placenta. Only after Shivers used dilators on her cervix, scraped out the uterine cavity, and washed it out with bichloride of mercury did the woman stop bleeding.[61] This case proved to Shivers, and probably to the family involved, that intrusive action saved the lives of miscarrying women. Doctors repeatedly reported in medical journals of miscarriage cases that involved great pain, profuse bleeding, fevers, and even "cataleptic trance."[62] By the 1880s, such reports also proved the success of intrusive action to decrease such dangerous symptoms.

Medical periodicals of the late nineteenth century also included accounts of women who were struck down with tetanus, convulsions, and even death in the wake of a miscarriage.[63] To be sure, this does not represent every case of miscarriage, and probably not even the majority. Many women undoubtedly miscarried at home, with help from family or friends, and quickly recovered with no lasting effects. But these were not the cases that doctors saw. Families called for doctors only when miscarriage, a common and perhaps recognizable event to most women, became abnormal. When nature could not take care of it neatly and easily, when tissues got stuck, fevers spiked, and pain became unending, then a doctor seemed appropriate. It only makes sense then that as physicians attended more and more miscarriages, they began describing the event as one that was always dangerous, always requiring swift action, and always abnormal.

Physicians also realized how the treatment of miscarriage could benefit them professionally. Many doctors, like Lusk, recognized how impressive they could appear to patients when presumably saving their lives with miscarriage treatment. In 1854, physician A. I. Cummings instructed his colleagues reading the *Boston Medical and Surgical Journal* that studying miscarriage was so important because there was no situation more professionally dire or dangerous to a young, inexperienced practitioner then a miscarrying woman "*bleeding to death.*"[64] One physician even laid out the argument for intervention for the good of a physician's reputation: "If he wavers or hesitates it is quickly observed, and confidence is weakened or lost."[65] In an era when regular physicians were attempting to convince potential patients why their services were superior to those of alternative practitioners who might have provided gentler and cheaper treatments or why a male physician was better suited to attend to pregnancy and childbirth than a female midwife, miscarriage became another battleground that could increase business and social standing for individual practitioners and improve the national reputation for the field as a whole.

In the middle of the century, physicians often relied on the wisdom of nature, but by the 1880s, they were much more likely to describe "her" as another inept practitioner. In 1891, Southern physician A. J. Swaney laid out his recommendations for miscarriage treatment, and while he did instruct others that "nature is ever to be given a chance," he quickly amended that advice: "but when we see her efforts are futile, certainly it is rational to assist her."[66] In his 1902 obstetrics text, Alexander Leuf cautioned his readers about emptying the uterus: "while nature will do this perfectly well most of the time if not interfered with, she sometimes does it as badly as it has so often been done by individuals."[67]

While continuing to reference the actions and duty of nature in cases of pregnancy loss, doctors altered their language when describing "her." In the middle of the nineteenth century, doctors argued that nature would do the job properly all on her own, whereas by the end of the century, doctors instead envisioned themselves as necessary to help nature, or even fix her mistakes. Doctors shifted the meaning of pregnancy loss from an event that was solely the work of nature to an event that required the combined efforts of medicine and nature, and then to an event that was more often successful because of medicine alone. We should also note how, as male physicians looked to discredit nature and promote their role in helping nature or fixing nature's mistakes, they repeatedly referred to nature as female. In an era when many of these same male physicians were involved in a struggle to stigmatize female midwives and run them out of business, it cannot be a coincidence that doctors also suggested that it was the ineptitude of another female figure that caused harm to reproducing women.

By the last two decades of the nineteenth century, American physicians seemed to agree that the best course of action in cases of miscarriage was immediate and intrusive action. Harvard gynecologist F. H. Davenport maintained in 1897 that one should not wait more than a few hours after the woman delivered the fetus before "interfering" and removing the placenta, while J. S. Baer promoted what perhaps could be seen as the rallying cry for the late nineteenth-century miscarriage treatment: "an empty uterus is a safe uterus, and the organ is only safe when it is empty."[68] This catchy slogan made sense when physicians were primarily seeing dangerous cases of miscarriage, not the ones with little pain, bleeding, and no fever. Physicians were responding to what they were encountering in the field: death by hemorrhage or septicemia as well as illnesses such as consumption from delayed action.[69] T. Gaillard Thomas claimed in 1890 that "vast numbers of women are invalided by abortion," while in 1870 William Byford asserted that "the effects of miscarriage upon the woman are almost always injurious."[70] Immediate cleaning out of the uterus forestalled the dramatic consequences of miscarriage that, for many physicians, seemed to be the only results of all miscarriage.

In an effort to improve intrusive actions and perhaps in a nod to their growing distrust of nature, physicians looked to metal instruments as the key to many of these treatments. In the early decades of the rise of intervention, however, doctors largely promoted the use of the finger to clean out the uterus. In 1858, William Tyler Smith warned against "instrumental devices" for removing the embryo, but he described using his finger "with time and patience" to bring away tissues.[71] Gunning S. Bedford claimed that instruments were "not only unnecessary but fraught with danger" and decided that the finger was the best extractor.[72] In 1864, Edward Spooner claimed "reliance on the finger is far safer and more satisfactory than any improvised hook or the best constructed small forceps."[73]

In the middle of the century, doctors' discussions of instruments in pregnancy-loss cases focused primarily on the instruments available: hooks, crochets, and forceps.[74] In 1866, the Obstetrical Society of London published their *Catalogue and Report of Obstetrical and Other Instruments*. In it, they claimed the two instruments utilized primarily for extraction of tissues in an abortion were forceps and hooks. Forceps, such as Sir James Simpson's ovum forceps, were between ten and fourteen inches long and typically resembled a pair of scissors, but with curved blades, either open, as in the case of Simpson's, or closed, for grasping onto the fetal tissue.[75] The catalog also included a description of a crotchet, which could be used to hook tissues and pull them out.[76]

Beginning in the 1880s, the curette quickly became the popular choice for those doctors on the lookout for instrumental aid in cases of pregnancy loss. The 1874 edition of the Matthews Brothers catalog of surgical instruments included various types of hooks, forceps, and dilators, but no curettes.[77] In contrast, the 1899 catalog of William Hatteroth's Surgical House in San Francisco contained eight different types of curettes.[78]

Curettes proved quite popular in discussions of the treatment of pregnancy loss in the last two decades of the nineteenth century. In his 1887 publication, *A Sketch of the Management of Pregnancy, Parturition and the Puerperal*, Paul Mundé, a New York physician and former editor of the *American Journal of Obstetrics*, recommended emptying the uterus at once with a large, dull curette.[79] Mundé was such a proponent for this method that some physicians identified him as the inventor of the curette.[80] In 1889, F. H. Davenport favored the sharp curette for scraping when pieces of tissue proved too small to be grasped with forceps.[81] By 1900, many doctors, such as David James Evans, were calling for thorough "curettement" in all cases of miscarriage.[82] Numerous other doctors supported the use of the curette, both in theory and in practice, toward the end of the nineteenth century.[83] Some also became involved in creating new and improved curettes for the multitudes of pregnancy-loss cases they faced. In 1898, Chicago doctor E. D. St Cyr introduced his version of the curette, a twisted instrument (resembling a corkscrew) that served "to propel the uterine contents downward and outward by simple external rotation and slight traction at its handle."[84]

By the turn of the twentieth century, American doctors seemed to be in agreement about the usefulness of the curette. In 1897, Wisconsin physician Mila Sharp argued that, while the curette had once been considered by the medical field as barbaric, opinion had changed, and with modifications, the instrument had become perfectly safe; indeed, with so many curettes to choose from, "none of the up-to-date physicians could consider his or her instrument-case complete without some, if not all of them."[85] In 1901, Henry Fry claimed that there was no question of the indications for the use of curette in cases of retained tissues in pregnancy loss.[86]

Conclusion

In May 1895, a forty-three-year-old married housewife came to the New England Hospital for Women and Children for help. Seven months pregnant, she reported that the pregnancy had gone well until about four weeks prior, when she started having convulsions. While having convulsions would seem like a good reason for anyone to visit a hospital today, in the late nineteenth-century many physicians reported treating this pregnancy symptom at home; indeed, hospitals at that time had no special equipment or medicines to better treat the affliction. A clue into why the woman came to the hospital in this instance may be her report that she had six children and had suffered five miscarriages. This was a woman experienced in reproduction, who seemingly had many failed attempts outside of the hospital.[87] Four months later, another married housewife, this one thirty-eight years old, came to the hospital when her waters broke in the sixth or seventh month of her pregnancy. While she admitted to no pain or bleeding—the hallmarks of miscarriage for most patients coming to the NEH—she may have better understood the significance, and danger, of her waters breaking than many women. This woman had been pregnant six times, but she gave birth only once at full term.[88]

The cases of these two women, and those of many others who came to the NEH in the final decade of the nineteenth century, reveal the success doctors had in convincing women and families that medicine could possibly be useful in the event of a miscarriage. In the first year of the maternity ward at NEH, around 17 percent of the women admitted reported having at least one miscarriage in their past. At its peak in 1898, this number rose to almost 27 percent.[89] As the century came to a close, more women with histories of miscarriage arrived at the NEH; perhaps they were looking for a new solution to their reproductive failures. Where Abigail Adams had bemoaned the ineptitude of physicians a century before, Boston women at the end of the 1800s saw potential value in the work of doctors in miscarriage cases.

Although it is perhaps easy to see the development of intrusive treatment of miscarriage in the latter decades of the nineteenth century as a physician-led and physician-benefiting enterprise, the evidence of women who flocked to the NEH, many other such institutions, and doctors in private practice also compels us to understand this development as one shaped by reproducing women themselves. Some of this shaping was indirect, because of the groups of women seeking medical help. When poor, working, immigrant, and single women appealed to physicians for aid, those doctors often determined that such patients did not deserve the same consideration and care, or even basic respect, that they doled out to wealthier patients. In 1897, Dr. J. A. Baughman visited the home of Mrs. J. M., who was seven months pregnant and "losing her waters." According to Baughman's report, Mrs. M. had been coming down a set of stairs with a child in one arm and a loaded rifle in the other, when she "dropped the weapon in such a manner as to discharge it, the ball entering her right thigh . . . [and] through the broad ligament into the uterus and amniotic sac." In his description, Baughman was not shy about expressing his disdain for his patient: "although American born, she belonged to the race of the great unwashed." Baughman delivered the dead fetus and the woman quickly recovered. After fifteen days, Mrs. M. was back to her household duties. Baughman closed his report on the case as follows: "If some of our city gentry who are engaged in checking over-population are on the *qui vive* [lookout] for something new I advise them to try a gun," suggesting, essentially, that lesser-valued groups of citizens should simply be shot.[90]

But women had a more direct role in this medical transformation as well—they actively sought out physicians and could use these new methods for their own design. In September 1895, a forty-three-year-old woman came to the NEH for a premature birth, but surprisingly, this was not an unexpected event. This Scottish housewife had experienced four miscarriages and two stillbirths and was looking for a way to make this pregnancy successful. She had arranged earlier to come to NEH in her eighth month to have her labor induced because, as nurses recorded, "she had never given birth to a living child." Doctors ruptured her membranes and she slept through the night. The next morning nurses provided hot douches, and by 9 P.M. the patient's pains had become severe and dilation was complete. Her baby, weighing 3 pounds, 14 ounces and measuring 46 centimeters in length, was born an hour later. Almost four weeks later, she was discharged, with the note: "baby strong and well; weighs 5 pounds 14 ounces."[91]

Between 1870 and 1900, according to reports in medical journals, American physicians attended an increasing number of miscarriage cases, and according to teaching texts and domestic health guides, they strongly urged women and families that all cases of pregnancy loss required medical attention. In response to the social and economic changes that brought poor and immigrant women to their doors, doctors began to see value in attending miscarriage cases. Women also saw value in including doctors in these experiences. Together women and doctors crafted miscarriage as an abnormal event, one that went against nature, a medical phenomenon that brought a healthy pregnancy to an unhealthy end. However, as it turns out, the greatest value to physicians in reframing miscarriage as abnormal and dangerous lay not in the increased business or professional status they could achieve through scraping out a woman's uterus. The greatest value of miscarriage was not in how it took away a pregnancy, but rather in how it produced a scientific specimen: the fetus.

5

The Body in the Clot

Medical Interest in Miscarried Tissues, 1870–1912

Born in Boston to a wealthy merchant, Caroline Healey grew up in a household of private tutors, Unitarian liberalism, and diverse intellectual influences. At the age of twelve, she attended lectures by Ralph Waldo Emerson and wrote summaries of them at the order of her father. She also often found herself running the family household and caring for her seven siblings during her mother's frequent illnesses. Early in life she began reform work, publishing in her teens on abolition and women's rights. In the wake of the Panic of 1837, a financial crisis in the United States that touched off a recession that lasted well into the 1840s, the Healey family's economic situation took a downturn, and Caroline began teaching to help sustain the family. She married Charles Dall, a young minister, in 1844, but the couple was soon living in her parents' house with their young son, William, because of her husband's inability to support them financially. In March 1847, Caroline Dall experienced her first miscarriage. Three months after disclosing her pregnancy in her diary, she wrote, "at—eleven o'clock A.M. began to flow . . . slept soundly through the night, but the flow was immense and became so copious and exhausting a stream, that I sent for Dr. Cheever. He presupposed a miscarriage [and] ordered me flat upon my back."[1] Almost exactly one year later, Dall again gave birth prematurely. This time, though, in her eighth month of

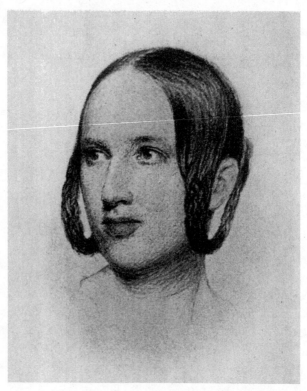

FIG. 7. Caroline Healey Dall (undated). (Collection of the Massachusetts Historical Society)

pregnancy, she described in detail her lost child, five weeks after the event: "My child! why should I call it so -! but after one has borne a second life about with her, for eight months—it is impossible not to love it, though it should prove an abortion." The child bore physical abnormalities, "no thumb on the right hand—but instead five fingers—the fifth growing out of the first. The smaller intestines were formed on the outside and the scrotum was deficient."[2]

When she first miscarried, perhaps sometime in her third or fourth month of pregnancy, Dall did not describe what had come out of her body, or what had become of the tissues. In contrast, when she gave birth to her almost full-term child, she described it in detail and recounted that her husband "buried his little one, with his own trembling hands."[3] Dall's latter pregnancy produced a child that was virtually full term, and therefore, regardless of its appearance, warranted burial. The body expelled in her earlier miscarriage perhaps warranted something different, but what?

An 1895 meeting of the Detroit Medical and Library Association begins to answer that question. On February 18, doctors from around the state of Michigan gathered to share new discoveries, discuss interesting cases, and commiserate over troublesome patients. The meeting opened, as was tradition, with an exhibition of specimens—a sort of medical show-and-tell. Dr. Theodore McGraw went first: "I have here a leg which I amputated for an old trouble of femur and knee-joint." He showed his audience evidence of osteo-myelitis, gelatinous degeneration, and erosion of the cartilage of the knee-joint, and an inflammatory condition of the tibia. In short, this was no normal leg. It was not merely the end product of an amputation, but one that gave visible, difficult-to-obtain evidence of multiple pathologies. Next up was a Dr. Hoyt, who simply stated: "I was called to deliver Mrs. S. I found her in labor at the full period. After delivering her of a normal child, I found this small fetus (about three inches long). It is nothing unusual except that the placenta was oblong."[4]

Dr. Hoyt helps us uncover the second half to the medical story of miscarriage. As physicians became more and more involved in the treatment of miscarriage and its complications, they often walked away from such cases with the resulting material products. By the end of the nineteenth century, women like Caroline Dall, who were more likely to call for a doctor when experiencing "flooding" during pregnancy, were also responsible for handing over the fetal and placental tissues that came out of their bodies. Perhaps initially this was an unintended consequence of the increase in medical attention to miscarriage, but physicians found themselves in possession of tiny beings, beings they discovered to be scientifically and socially valuable.

As the influential German zoologist Ernst Haeckel, who was professor of comparative anatomy at the University of Jena at the time, pronounced in an 1874 textbook, "human embryos conceal a greater wealth of important truths and form a more abundant source of knowledge than is afforded by the whole mass of most other sciences and of all so-called 'revelations' put together."[5] We cannot, however, simply take Haeckel's words as sentiments shared by all scientists, nor can we make the assumption that the human fetus inherently carries some meaning of an authoritative or unmediated representation of human development; in fact, there are many sites for its production and interpretation.[6] Each of these sites—be they bedrooms, personal letters, medical offices, university lectures, or museum exhibits—help to construct the fetus into a socially situated object that fashions human development in complicated ways. To better understand how the fetus obtained the social and political power that it holds today, we need to better ascertain how each site and each actor involved in the nineteenth-century embryological endeavors of physicians and the medicalization of miscarriage ascribed a meaning on this new object, and why.[7]

One of the reasons for the intense medical attention given to miscarriage cases beginning in the second half of the nineteenth century was that these cases, while they might have been referred to as losses, ends, or partings, also produced something very important: a scientific specimen. American physicians at this time were so interested in these tissues that they altered their practices, lied to their patients, and went to great lengths to obtain, preserve, and share these new research objects with their fellow doctors. This chapter will investigate *why* miscarriage products proved so valuable to nineteenth-century American physicians. In so doing, it will also uncover the complex process physicians undertook to reconstruct miscarriage products into scientific specimens. By investigating these social and scientific endeavors, I hope to reveal that early characterization of the fetus as a scientific specimen helped to shape the public understanding and acceptability of fetal bodies in late nineteenth-century America and today.

In some sense, this chapter is about materiality. It asks the questions: What was the object, tissue, or body that was contained in pregnancy and expelled in miscarriage? How did people make sense of these materials, and why did they interpret them the way they did? To that end, this study reveals the multiple forces that created connections between bodies—both maternal and fetal—and social categories. By exploring the transfer of embryonic and fetal tissues from a family to a doctor, we can better understand the social influences on scientific knowledge.

Women and doctors worked together, sometimes for vastly different reasons, in coproducing embryological knowledge. Looking to better understand their miscarriage experiences within larger reproductive desires and abilities, many women freely handed over miscarriage products to the medical men at their bedsides, perhaps finding comfort in the transformation from pregnancy to specimen. In turn, the physicians who were seeking these specimens for clues to human development and the hidden science of pregnancy excitedly whisked specimens away from the bedside of their patients, studied them in offices, shared them at society meetings, and utilized them to answer questions about conception, gestation, and what it means to be human. A close analysis of this clinical interaction reveals the complexity of scientific discovery and highlights the role of women in the access to and meanings of fetal and embryonic specimens.[8]

Finding Bodies

In most histories of American human embryology, the story begins with Franklin P. Mall.[9] Born to German immigrants in Iowa, Mall graduated from the University of Michigan Medical School in 1883. Like most young doctors at the time, he immediately set off for further training in Europe with influential embryology researchers such as the Swiss anatomist Wilhelm His. One of the more celebrated figures in German embryology, His had accumulated a personal collection of almost eighty embryos, which he referred to as "treasures," and he was gaining fame for his solid fixing techniques of the specimens. Mall returned to the United States in 1886, equipped with two small human embryos he received as a gift from His, and immediately set out to amass a large collection of human embryos and fetuses. Utilizing all of his professional and medical connections, Mall appealed to the wider American medical community to send any and all fetal and embryonic specimens to him for cataloging, preserving, and study. His hard work paid off with the establishment of the Carnegie Institute Department of Embryology in 1914, which became a new institutional home for Mall's 813 specimens and the site for the emergence of American dominance in human embryology.[10] What scholars tend to neglect in this narrative is that Mall's success in specimen collecting hinged on the presence of a medical community that had already been interested in collecting fetal specimens for decades. Investigating the American medical tradition of fetal collection in the years prior to Mall's institutionalization of the practice not only extends the story back in time, but it also reveals the women who are embedded in each discovery, published article, and professional presentation.[11]

While nineteenth-century European university-based embryologists and anatomists certainly ignored the women who physically produced the needed specimens and often disregarded the work of physicians who initially collected them, historians should not do likewise and discount these two groups in the history of this emerging science.[12] Nineteenth-century embryology was not an enterprise restricted to European laboratories and universities, as is too often portrayed in the historiography. American physicians, both country practitioners and esteemed urban professors, collected miscarriage products in attempts to learn more about the curious development of a human being. This study seeks to acknowledge the role of doctors in early embryology as well as to consider how and why practitioners gained access to these newly valued specimens.[13] Women's attitudes about miscarriage, and reproduction more generally, were essential to the emergence of this new field of study that was created by doctors who were allowed to take miscarriage materials away from the bedside.[14] Integral to this analysis of the role of women is the reminder that in the second half of the nineteenth century, most medical care, including childbirth, took place in the home. This physical location gave women, and their female attendants and families, more power over the doctors intruding upon the domestic realm.[15]

As discussed before, the shift in medical and philosophical thinking from preformation to epigenesis altered the very identity of the tissues expelled in miscarriage. In the early nineteenth century, doctors primarily understood human development to be intensely interesting, but largely unavailable for research. In Samuel Bard's popular 1819 midwifery text, the New York physician and professor included a general description of the developing embryo, including circulation, anatomy of the umbilical cord, and the appearance of each major organ in development. But Bard very clearly pointed out to his students that the "opportunities for observing the progress of the human embryo, with the same exactness and particularity with which it has been investigated in other animals, never can be obtained."[16] In 1832, noted American obstetrician William Potts Dewees agreed, claiming that while "a strong and certainly laudable curiosity is almost always felt by the students, to ascertain the progress of development of the foetus," in fact, "knowledge upon this subject must necessarily be both limited and uncertain."[17] In the first few decades of the nineteenth century, American physicians showed a marked interest in human development, but they also viewed it as a subject that was largely beyond the limits of what was knowable. Unlike the chick, which biologists could experiment on and sacrifice at will, the human embryo was simply not available for such study, in no small part because miscarriage cases more often resulted in "bubbly lots" than in discernible embryos.

By the 1830s, references to fruit, chaos, and other strange objects that were so often expelled in cases of miscarriage faded away in medical writings and were replaced by a sense of awe at the marvels of human development available for scrutiny at the bedside of a miscarrying woman. Under epigenesis, those amorphous masses that slipped from women's bodies through miscarriage could be reconstructed to represent normal human development. "Fleshy morsels" were now human embryos or fetuses, ready specimens that provided insights into human life and death.[18]

Only thirteen years after Dewees asserted that embryology was limited and uncertain, a Dr. Lopez elevated the status of a misshapen and contaminated four-month fetus from routine discharges to a compelling scientific specimen. In March 1839, Lopez had been summoned to attend "Louisa, a coloured woman," or, more specifically, to attend what had come out of her uterus. Two days after Louisa delivered a healthy child with a midwife in attendance, the women caring for her decided to call in Dr. Lopez to help identify a newly discovered object "which had been thrust aside unobserved, on the day of parturition, among the soiled clothing and discharges." Lopez quickly determined the object to be an interesting specimen, a small fetus, and took it away for further investigation.[19]

Intrigued by the small body, Lopez took the fetus away from Louisa's bedside and house and placed it in a bottle of alcohol for preservation. He then attempted to transport the specimen from South Carolina to Alabama in order to present his treasure before the Medical Society of Mobile. Along the way the bottle broke, the alcohol evaporated, and mold soon covered the entire surface of the fetus. Then while attempting to clean the specimen, Lopez inadvertently detached the umbilical cord, effectively ruining an important aspect of the specimen: the coiling of the cord around one knee and thigh. Even in its moldy and damaged state, this small body became the topic of a lengthy discussion at the meeting and ultimately a twenty-two-page article on a variety of subjects, including the necessity of female orgasm for successful conception, the origin and preserving powers of amniotic fluid, and the possibility of spontaneous amputation within the womb.[20]

Dr. Lopez was not the only American physician to focus miscarriage case reports on the fate of the products rather than the recovery of the patient, and he was far from the only practitioner to show up at a medical society meeting with an ovum or fetus in hand. By the 1850s, midwifery and obstetric texts no longer lamented the limits of scientific knowledge when it came to human development. In comparison to the scant twelve pages Dewees devoted to the subjects of the membranes, placenta, and fetal circulation, an 1858 publication, *The Principles and Practice of Obstetrics*, by Henry Miller, a professor of obstetric medicine at the University of Louisville, reveals quite a different attitude. In his text, spread across forty-nine pages, Miller described the decidua, provided a very detailed analysis of amniotic fluid (including its taste), and included a detailed chronicle of the anatomical developments of the embryo.[21]

Physicians gained new confidence in the possibility of studying embryology in practice as well. In 1871, Dr. E. Chenery was called in to attend a woman, five months pregnant, who was bleeding and in great pain. As he later disclosed: "she had passed nearly a chamber-vessel full of blood and clots, among which I found a foetus . . . of about the size of a common open-faced watch."[22] Not only did Chenery believe that he could see something in the blood and clots, but he valued the specimen enough to dig through a chamber pot full of them. A century earlier, physicians would have been expected to interpret these clots as only clots, or possibly a product of false conception.

In theory, physicians had multiple avenues available to them for gaining access to fetal specimens, including autopsies of pregnant women, surgical procedures (like hysterectomy), and abortions. However, with the availability of pregnant female bodies for autopsy (or really, any bodies) severely limited, major gynecological surgeries such as hysterectomies still posing dire threats of mortality through infection, and more and more states outlawing abortion between the 1850s and 1880s, attending a miscarriage proved to be the most viable path to obtaining fetal tissues—a path that could be at once accessible to physicians and assured of specimen success.[23] Miscarriage, perceived as a frequent occurrence among women who spent as many as forty years reproducing, allowed doctors of all types a chance to investigate the wonders of the human body without social or professional consequences.

Collecting Bodies

Before physicians could fully integrate fetal tissues into the world of scientific research, they first needed to negotiate the transfer of these specimens away from their female patients and sometimes other female attendants. This new location for fetal collection could be a space of despair, relief, or subterfuge, but more compellingly, it could also be a site of collaboration between women and doctors. Early medical investigation into human development depended on the intimate clinical encounter necessary to the production of these specimens. Women and their families played a key role in embryologic knowledge production through deciding what tissues might have been (fetus, child, clot, or something else) and what was to be done with them. In every case of miscarriage, a woman and perhaps her husband and/or other family members made a decision about what to do with the "stuff" that came out. Most women's writings about pregnancy loss give little clue to what happened to the resulting materials. It is probably the case that some materials were buried, and archeological evidence suggests some were discarded in privies or other disposal sites, but medical sources reveal another fate of fetal tissues—their entry into the world of research. Many of these tissues ended up in the hands, offices, and societies of American doctors, and the initial power to put them in those hands rested with American families.

For physicians lucky enough to be included in miscarriage cases, the resulting specimens proved to be quite valuable. In 1884, a Dr. Hendrix brought what he dubbed "an interesting specimen" to the St. Louis Medical Society: a fetus "thrown off" in the seventh month and still within the placenta. The doctors gathered at the meeting agreed with Hendrix that it was unusual to find a late-term fetus with sack and cord so complete. Hendrix admitted that while he usually attempted to arrive at a case before labor was complete, this time he benefited from his tardiness because it kept him from rupturing the membranes, a common practice to ease a patient and speed up labor. Instead, by not following his typical procedure, Hendrix ended up with an almost magical object. Holding the specimen in front of the group, Hendrix demonstrated its value, stating, "I can turn the foetus almost into any position whilst in the sac."[24]

Hendrix does not inform us of what his patient thought of his removing the materials from her home, but it is quite possible that she readily handed them over. Not every physician was so fortunate, and a few complained of this power the family held over the fate of miscarriage products. In 1880, Alex Y. P. Garnett, then emeritus professor of clinical medicine at the National Medical College of the District of Columbia, published a case of miscarriage in the *American Journal of the Medical Sciences*. Garnett was called in to attend a twenty-four-year-old woman suffering from uterine hemorrhage. The patient in question suspected she was pregnant, and upon careful examination, Garnett diagnosed "pregnancy with accidental haemorrhage." Eventually Garnett determined that miscarriage was inevitable, and he stayed by her bed for the next twenty-four hours. Finally, the woman passed a five-month-old fetus, and Garnett reported of his desire to fully examine the specimen, but wrote: "I regret to say that this was necessarily limited to a mere inspection and manipulation of the foetus and its environments, as I was not permitted to remove the specimen from the house, thereby depriving me of an auxiliary examination by the microscope." Garnett did not explain who refused him further access or on what grounds. He did, however, take the time to make a sketch of the specimen for inclusion in his published article.[25]

In 1892, Dr. T. R. Rubush presented a similar case before the Indiana State Medical Society. Rubush attended a young woman suffering intense bearing-down pain and hemorrhage in her sixth month of pregnancy. Soon after, she delivered twins, which Rubush determined to be between the fourth and fifth month of development. After describing the twins in glowing and fascinated language, Rubush disclosed, "I made an earnest effort to secure the children ... to preserve as specimens, but failed, the parents objecting to it."[26]

A few doctors described the lengths they went to in order to circumvent this family power altogether. In 1859, Ohio physician James Irvine attended the labor of a "Mrs. S, aged 22, a stout, healthy looking woman." Expecting a full-term birth, Irvine was surprised, upon examination, to find a premature fetus presenting. Once it emerged, Irvine reported, "This I concealed under the bed-clothes, informing my patient and the bystanders that it was merely the passage of a few clots of blood." Irvine continued to deliver the expected full-term infant and then "directed the all-inquisitive nurse to go down stairs and make the mother a cup of tea, and during her absence [he] ascertained that the mass first expelled was a foetus of from four to five months, in a high state of preservation."[27] A Dr. Atchison reported of a similar doing in an 1868 edition of the *American Journal of the Medical Sciences*. Called in to attend a case of miscarriage at seven months, Atchison was surprised to find, in addition to the expected fetus, a second one of about four months gestation. In considering the woman's report of possible causes of the miscarriage, Atchison informed his audience, "It must be remembered that the mother does not know of the second fetus," indicating some sort of deception.[28]

This possibility of taking fetal specimens was reflected in the language of some case reports as well. In 1840, Maryland physician William Zollickoffer recounted a case of an interesting miscarriage in which he delivered one fetus and two placentas. At the end of the account, Zollickoffer stated, "I have regretted exceedingly, since the occurrence of this circumstance, that I had not pocketed the curious productions for preservation in alcohol."[29] It is telling that Zollickoffer used the term "pocketed" in referring to how he would have removed the tissues. Rather than simply taking the specimen with him when he left, Zollickoffer imagined he would have had to be sneaky, to hide it in a pocket perhaps. Whether or not Zollickoffer actually imagined putting the fetal tissues in his coat pocket, the language he chose does indicate that he considered the action may have carried some sort of deception.

While physicians' reports of family resistance to the medical removal of miscarriage products prove to be a minority in the medical literature, these few cases do reveal that not all American families understood fetal remains to be waste products with little value. Some retained the tissues involved in miscarriage to bury or burn, perhaps viewing the clots as family members or personal property. Caroline Dall, after all, reported the burial of her premature birth.[30] Although scholars have described the historical status of fetal tissues primarily in terms of waste, the medical reports and personal writings such as Dall's reveal the variety of ways

Americans interpreted miscarriage products. Some tissues certainly ended up in chamber pots and possibly even privies, but others remained valued possessions.[31]

Doctors valued and desired these new specimens enough to lie to patients, but also enough to alter their practice. In 1896, Detroit physician Dr. William Stevens presented four specimens to the Michigan State Medical Society. In the case of the third specimen, Stevens revealed that when he first examined the patient, he "found the sack protruding from the os." However, "wishing to procure the specimen intact, the case was left to nature."[32] Whether or not Stevens knew about or agreed with the numerous medical publications of the time warning against leaving a miscarriage to nature (because it left the woman at risk of hemorrhage and sepsis), it is striking that his actions (or lack of) were driven by his hopes of obtaining a specimen, rather than by the needs of his patient.[33]

The intense interest in, and the value placed on fetal tissues reveals how the inclusion of pregnancy loss into the story of the medicalization of reproduction complicates our existing interpretation. Historians commonly look to regular doctors' aim to gain a monopoly over the marketplace, desires to stem the falling fertility rates of the white middle class, and responses to consumer demand all as reasons for the increased male medical oversight of pregnancy, birth, and infertility in the late nineteenth and early twentieth centuries.[34] An investigation into miscarriage, however, reveals the role of scientific specimens in this medicalization movement. Some of the impetus for doctors to rush to the bedsides of pregnant and birthing women was that they might have a chance to obtain these tiny objects—portable enough to put in your pocket and yet magnificent enough to provide a wealth of information about the science of man.

In 1885, J. H. Etheridge exhibited a four-month-old fetus with placenta before the Chicago Gynecological Society. The society found the specimen extremely interesting, both in its appearance (it was extremely flattened) and in the fact that it was delivered immediately in the wake of the birth of a full-term infant. Much discussion about the process of conception and the role of the placenta in nutrition followed Etheridge's exhibition. Professor Daniel T. Nelson even thought "it would be interesting to know how much force was necessary to compress the foetus" in such a way and referred to the experiments of Professor Park of the Massachusetts Agricultural College, who worked on determining the expansile force of growing squashes and pumpkins.[35]

Unfortunately, human fetuses were not pumpkins. Scientists could not test how much force was required to compress a fetus. Physicians and biologists were limited to looking for snapshots of human development in the fetal tissues produced by cases of pregnancy loss. Even in the face of the advent of experimental embryology at the end of the nineteenth century, these valued tissues remained the primary method for investigating the creation of humans, and doctors found themselves on the front lines of these scientific explorations.

Physicians also valued miscarriage products as scientific markers. Obtaining these tissues was a way for physicians with no access to laboratories or expensive equipment (or cadavers) to participate in the larger enterprise of crafting American medicine into scientific medicine. In 1872, Dr. Cephas L. Bard was living and practicing in San Buenaventura, California (now Ventura), a small frontier town far from the academic halls of the Eastern universities that were housing the debates on the utility of basic sciences in medical education, and further still from the "science" coming out of European labs and hospitals. But when Bard came across a three-month-old fetus in his practice, he could conduct scientific research on the object and enter into an international conversation about the science of human development.[36] In an era when mainstream doctors sought ways to create a public image suffused with validity and professionalism and viewed science as a way to do that, having a human fetus in one's office could be extremely helpful.

Partial Deaths and Small Cadavers

In order to fully understand why physicians valued miscarried fetal tissues so much in the second half of the nineteenth century, I want to focus on two major debates within the medical literature: how to determine and understand the processes of life and death; and the possibility of superfetation. While nineteenth-century physicians from all over the country and from many different backgrounds utilized miscarried fetuses to determine causes of miscarriage, the mechanics of conception and fetal development, and how the amniotic sac actually worked, larger social and professional changes at the time also drove these practitioners to view fetal tissues as special answers to understanding the process of life. In an era of transforming views of death and the dead body through domestication, commodification, and photographic visualization, doctors valued the human fetus—not only as a unique object for investigating the process of death but also as a handy stand-in for unavailable adult cadavers.[37]

By the 1870s and 1880s, Americans had a wholly new and complicated relationship to death. During the Civil War, many Americans faced death on a daily basis, often forced to contend with the vast quantities of dead bodies surrounding them, both in person and through the new technology of photography.[38] At the same time, the emerging middle class used the management of death to help sustain and exhibit gentility. New mourning practices, including death portraits, the rural cemetery movement, and the importance of proper mourning attire, all helped to create a new social meaning for death.[39] At the same time, doctors struggled to obtain dead bodies for use in medical teaching and research—a largely futile enterprise. Within this larger context, miscarriage provided doctors an alternative path into understanding how humans live and die.

In 1866, Dr. J. Stolz attended the miscarriage of sixteen-year-old Mrs. B, who delivered "a living female foetus, at about the fifth month of uterine gestation." Stolz cut the umbilical cord, wrapped the fetus in flannel and laid it on the sofa, returning to his patient to attend to her hemorrhage. Once he deemed her safe, he turned his attention back to the fetus, and to his surprise found it still alive, gasping for breath. He described the fetus as follows: "Pulsation could be felt and seen in the thorax and fontanelles. Life continued for some time, even after I had carried it to my office, where it was also witnessed by my professional friends, Drs. Booth and Jenners. It gradually succumbed, after surviving its birth one hour and forty minutes. It measured about six inches in length."[40] Mrs. B's miscarriage provided Dr. Stolz with a unique research object—a live human, or at least human body that he could remove from the family, share with colleagues, and upon which he could closely observe the complex pathway from life to death.

This interest in the fetus is more understandable when we remember that by the end of the nineteenth century, doctors were convinced of the value of studying physiology and anatomy but also faced legal and social strictures limiting their access to the human cadavers needed for these studies. The fetus served as a handy stand-in for the cadaver. It could still illuminate much about the workings of the human body, but without the moral tensions of cutting open someone's dead family member. There was the added bonus, of course, that fetuses were small enough to put in your pocket.

These small objects, portable and yet extraordinary, could provide information about how certain systems worked, how a body could die, and unlike adult cadavers, some could even be available still alive. In 1898, a case out of Europe caught the eyes of the publishers of the New York University Medical School journal, the *Post-Graduate*. In it, Dr. Franz Neugebauer reported of operating on a case of extrauterine pregnancy. He described, in graphic detail, dismembering the fetus, including penetrating the skull, in order to remove it, and he ended the report by noting "the remarkable observation was made in this fetus that for several hours the heart action persisted," even after the head was torn off with the entire spinal cord. In this case, Neugebauer could utilize a fetus to better understand the motions of the heart, and its connections to other systems of the body, in a violent manner that would have been unthinkable on an adult, or meaningless on a cadaver.

The second half of the nineteenth century was also a time when some American physicians were very interested in working out the boundaries of life, especially in terms of the unborn. Horatio Storer, an esteemed Boston physician, began his national crusade against abortion in the late 1850s, and he published copiously about how the practice was equivalent to infanticide. In his widely debated and influential writings supporting the illegalization of abortion at any time during pregnancy, Storer claimed that the human fetus could exist only in one of two states—life or death—and if not one, then it must be the other.[41] However, this construct of fetal life had strikingly little influence on the broader medical literature. Despite Storer's credentials, his arguments about fetal life did not influence thinking about miscarriage or even pregnancy more broadly in medical periodicals or teaching texts, even if they did prove to be highly successful in changing legislation.[42]

While Storer and a handful of his fellow academic physicians espoused rhetoric that painted embryos and fetuses as alive as fully grown adults, many doctors felt little hesitation at interpreting the products of miscarriage outside of a stark life–death binary. These physicians instead conceptualized the products of miscarriage as existing as alive and dead at the same time, focusing on the tissues as valuable clues to the very categories of life and death. In 1850, Dr. S. B. Davis of Franklin County, Ohio, found himself attending a curious case of pregnancy loss when he was called to attend a woman in labor in the seventh month of her pregnancy. After the fetus and placenta were delivered without much trouble, Davis discovered the sac of another fetus. He was surprised to discover that "the second fetus proved to be of about six weeks growth [and] its whole appearance was fresh, without a sign of putrefaction."

Davis wondered how, what he called "the minor foetus," could lose its "vitality," but not decay within the womb where it had remained for so long. He consulted with other doctors, one who suggested that the growing fetus "imparts a *something* to the lifeless ovum, sufficient to counteract the effects of the putrefactive process." Davis was not satisfied with this explanation and felt that the key to solving the mystery was that not only was the minor fetus kept fresh, but that *"its vessels were patulous and contained blood."* Davis concluded that circulation between the mother and the fetus had continued until the delivery, but something had affected the supply of blood to diminish it "to such a degree as to check its growth and development; yet enough remaining to keep in a little life."[43] Davis viewed this product of miscarriage as a boundary object in the life–death binary. It contained "a little life," enough life to keep the fetus fresh and prevent decomposition, but not enough to sustain its development into a full-term child.

Alex Garnett echoed this idea that life and death could exist in quantities in his 1880 article in the *American Journal of the Medical Sciences*. Garnett was called in to attend a pregnant woman with slight uterine hemorrhage and ended up treating her for the next month. Finally, she delivered a five-month-old fetus, about which Garnett reported: "contrary to my expectations, [it] gave unmistakable evidence of feeble vitality." Garnett examined the fetus and sac carefully, looking for the cause "which had finally culminated in the partial death and expulsion of the foetus."[44] While the miscarriage products showed some "vitality," they did not yet constitute a fully alive body or individual. Products of miscarriage, for doctors, occupied a liminal space between life and death: not yet born and yet sometimes bodies that breathed, pulsed, moved, or cried. They could be a little alive, or partially dead.

In a culture preoccupied with the changing reality and meaning of death, nineteenth-century doctors looked to products of miscarriage not only to give clues about the distinction, or lack thereof, between the categories of life and death, but also to provide insights into how humans actually died. Death in nineteenth-century America was still a very domestic event, dealt with by family, friends, neighbors, and religious advisors rather than any sort of medical professionals.[45] Doctors were often not allowed entry to this personal, family event, and thus they had little opportunity to closely observe a human body in the process of passing from life to death, beyond that of their own family members. Miscarriage products, however, allowed physicians the chance to observe and research death in a way that was much more socially acceptable than would have been for adult bodies.

In 1852, Dr. A. W. Barrows presented a case before the Hartford Medical Association. After attending a woman in her fifth month of pregnancy, Barrows departed with a live fetus, completely encased in its sac, for further study. He described finally rupturing the membranes upon which the fetus uttered a cry, and he continued to note its condition: it breathed for forty minutes, it stuck its tongue out at various intervals, it made occasional voluntary movements of the extremities, and its heart beat for three-quarters of an hour.[46] Barrows kept watch over the fetus, as he said, "with interest and care," but he did not describe attempts to aid with respiration, keep it warm, or any other life-saving techniques common at the time for premature births. Instead, he simply observed it, much like one would an exotic insect. Barrows's study of this fetus gave him a keen glimpse into the very processes that made one dead or alive, without the moral implications of removing a dying child from its family or home.

This intermediate status of miscarriage products is perhaps mostly clearly exhibited in the case of Charles Munde, one of the leaders in the hydrotherapy movement. In 1849, Munde emigrated from Dresden to New York, with the notion of setting up a water-cure practice in Baltimore. Hailed by the *New York Tribune* as "next to Priessnitz, the most eminent practitioner of Water-Cure that Germany has produced," Munde and his wife arrived on American shores in a moment of personal trauma.[47] When they set out, Munde's wife was pregnant, but according to her husband, the stress of "the German Revolution . . . the parting with her friends, the cholera, [and] the sea voyage" was all too much for her pregnant body. She miscarried in her fifth month soon after arriving in America, with her husband providing medical aid. Munde described the events in an 1850 article, and after a lengthy account of his wife's ordeals, he closed the piece with: "After twenty-two hours from the beginning of the accident, the foetus, a boy (whom I preserve in alcohol) went off."[48] In this liminal space of both medical encounter and personal disappointment, Munde viewed the fetus as something that was more appropriate in a jar of alcohol than in hallowed ground. One cannot help but wonder if his wife ever saw the jar or what she thought of it.

Superfetation

In addition to the valuable insights a miscarried fetus could provide physicians in terms of how humans lived and how they died, these tiny creatures could also prove useful in better understanding the changing racial landscape of late nineteenth-century America. Fetal tissues were biological proof of the need for increased social anxieties about and control over the proper separation of the races, via investigations into superfetation, or conception within an already pregnant woman. In the early nineteenth century doctors relied on the work of William Hunter to show the impossibility of superfetation. Hunter, a highly influential and well-known Scottish anatomist and obstetrician (perhaps best known for his large-scale illustrated atlas of pregnancy, *The Anatomy of the Gravid Uterus*, published in 1774), argued that almost immediately upon implantation of a fertilized egg, a closed sac formed on the inside of the uterus. Further, soon after implantation, a mucous plug formed in the cervix. These two physical barriers, the sac and the plug, prevented eggs from descending into the uterus, as well as sperm from entering via the cervix, thus putting a halt to any additional fertilizations.

By the middle of the nineteenth century, many researchers sought to disprove the great master. In 1842, the French physiologist Victor Coste presented the results of his investigations on the anatomy of the pregnant woman, which he obtained over a number of years and primarily carried out on the bodies of women who had committed suicide. In these results, Coste displayed images of two of his subjects: one from a woman in her eighth week of pregnancy, the other in the third month. Coste argued that it was apparent in these bodies that the uterus did not contain a closed sac, but instead contained two membranes—the decidua vera and the decidua reflexa—with a cavity in between. This space could allow sperm to travel into the uterus from the cervix, as well as meet up with eggs from the fallopian tubes.[49]

In his 1868 text, *Researches in Obstetrics*, British physician J. Matthews Duncan published results of microscopic studies on the mucous plug during pregnancy. Duncan argued that the mucous present during pregnancy was no different from the mucous present in a nonpregnant female.[50] With the evidence against both the mucous plug and the membrane separating the egg and sperm after conception, doctors also began to question the traditional notion that women did not menstruate during pregnancy. Overall, physicians indicated that while it was a general rule that menstruation ceased during pregnancy (and indeed it was often cited as a sign of pregnancy), most were unable to deny the clinical evidence that contradicted the rule. Thomas Hawkes Tanner claimed, "as a rule, a woman does not experience any menstrual discharge during gestation; yet no one denies that this is a rule to which there are many exceptions." He continued, "and as we sometimes see that the external signs of ovulation are manifested, why should we argue that those which are naturally unseen are absent?"[51] Once doctors and physiologists denounced both the plug and the closed sac, menstruation during pregnancy (deemed in the Hunterian tradition as highly pathologic and rare) could be reclassified both as possible and as natural. Duncan argued, "Menstruation proper is a generally-received indication that conception is possible. And there is no valid reason to believe that this does not hold equally good of the menstruation occurring in early pregnancy as at other times."[52]

By 1874, superfetation seemed so plausible that Gunning Bedford argued, "physiological research, aided by clever microscopists, has demonstrated that Hunter's view was little less than fiction," and that "there can be no doubt that two fecundations may take place within a very short period of each other."[53] Many physicians agreed with Bedford in support of both the clinical evidence for superfetation and its anatomical possibility.[54] Throughout the second half of the nineteenth century, more and more physicians published accounts of attending a woman for a normal labor, only to discover that, along with the full-term baby, the woman was also carrying a younger fetus.[55] Doctors also described attending cases of miscarriage and coming away with two specimens of different stages.[56] And some even depicted cases in which two full-term births took place within weeks of each other.[57] In 1882, Henry Allen of Hoboken, New Jersey, reported that after helping a patient control her hemorrhage in the wake of delivering a four-month fetus, upon his return a number of days later, he found she had passed a clot. He disclosed, "upon examining it closely, I discovered it to be another ovum, and, upon making an incision, to my surprise found another foetus within it. This I still have in my possession." Allen maintained that this case was clearly an example of superfetation.[58]

In contrast to the first half of the century, late nineteenth-century physicians generally agreed on the plausibility of superfetation, as well as its inherent interest. This debate, which continued into the first few decades of the twentieth century, was made possible by the collection of fetal tissues by physicians. Doctors, valuing the materials produced by miscarriage, began to "see" knowledge of human development in clots that previously would have been discounted as either only clots, or as not natural.

Some of the emerging interest in superfetation was a display of the superiority of modern obstetrics—with its scientific research and microscopic studies—over blindly following a Hunterian tradition. But in many of these reported cases of possible superfetation (and there were a surprising number) physicians also referred to a much older case for support. In his famous work, *Natural History*, eighteenth-century French naturalist and mathematician Georges Louis Leclerc, comte de Buffon, related a story of a woman in Charleston, South Carolina, who in 1714 gave birth to two children, one immediately after the other. As Buffon described: "To the utter astonishment of all present, one child was black and the other white. From the evident testimony of her infidelity to her husband, the woman acknowledged, that a negro had one day entered her chamber, where her husband had just left her in bed, and by threats of immediate death, compelled her to gratify his desires."[59]

Numerous physicians repeated this tale and frequently supplemented it with similar stories, as Samuel Bard did, in his widely referenced 1819 text on midwifery. Bard recounted a case of a white servant of Abington, Maryland, who delivered twins, "one of which was perfectly white, the other perfectly black." Dr. Bard professed of knowing these twins later in life and described the white girl as "delicate, fair skinned, light haired and blue eyed," whereas her sister "has all the characterizing marks of the African; short of stature, flat and broad nosed, thick lipped, woolly headed, flat footed, and projecting heels." Bard continued, "she is said to resemble a negro they had on the farm, but with whom the mother never would acknowledge an intimacy; but of this there was no doubt, as he and the white man, with whom her connexion was detected, both ran from the neighborhood, so soon as it was known the girl was with child."[60]

In 1849, Thomas Taylor reported to the *New York Journal of Medicine* on a similar case: "Clarissa, a negress, the property of Mr. A. Knox, aged about 35 years, in May last, was delivered of twins: one a mulatto, and the other a negro child." Apparently, Clarissa had intercourse with a white man three weeks after she felt she had conceived with her husband, with whom she had several children. Taylor claimed that at birth, "the mulatto child bore marks of being at least three weeks younger than the negro." This evidence convinced Taylor that the case was one of superfetation.[61]

As Philadelphia physician Dr. George Gould argued in 1900, "the most curious and convincing examples of superfetation are those in which children of different colors are born to the same woman."[62] New York physician Gunning Bedford labeled these sets of mixed-race twins "freaks of nature," and he was definitely not alone in viewing such cases of superfetation and the miscegenation (the sexual relations of or procreation between persons of perceived different races) involved as unnatural.[63] Physicians continued to use the Charleston case as proof of superfetation in the medical literature until at least 1921.[64] These cases proved so important and provocative because, first, they validated accepted sexual stereotypes: passive white female, violent and aggressive African American male, and adulterous and hypersexual African American female. Second, they mirrored Reconstruction concerns about black sexuality and how to properly separate the races without the institution of slavery. If superfetation was possible, the biological barrier to the production of these "freaks of nature" was removed, and thus surely society needed to step in to prevent further cases, necessitating legal and social strictures against practices such as miscegenation. The many cases of miscarried fetuses of different ages delivered simultaneously, or fetuses delivered alongside full-term infants, allowed physicians to authoritatively step in and help solve a pressing social problem.

Creating a Specimen

However much physicians valued miscarriage products, reconstructing them into scientific specimens was not a straightforward undertaking. Transforming the tissues that had previously stood as proof of pregnancy and represented the future of a family member into tissues integrated within scientific networks required some disentangling and reentangling work by physicians.[65] In order to interpret these bloody tissues and clots as research objects, physicians needed to integrate miscarriage products in scientific networks, and they did so in a variety of ways, sometimes all at once, but more commonly by creating science where and when they could.

One aim of this study is to expand our understanding of specimen-collection practices and their incorporated social meanings. In recent years historians and anthropologists have made steps to include the practice of collection within studies of the history of human sciences.[66] These studies, however, primarily focus on the work carried out on specimens in laboratories or other spaces of formal science. When the existence of specimens in the lab is not assumed, analysis of the initial site of transfer (from woman to doctor at her home) becomes essential. Thus, I analyze how women disentangled the tissues from their grounding in pregnancy and family and how physicians remade them into specimens and reentangled them into networks of scientific research.

The first step for many physicians in disentangling fetal tissues from a context of families and pregnancy was to remove them from the homes of their patients. If we look only to the presentations of miscarriage materials at professional gatherings or within the pages of medical journals, we miss out on half of the story. Dr. Lopez, after all, did not simply find his moldy specimen on the side of the road. In order for doctors to obtain these newly valued objects, women and their families needed to include medical attendants in their miscarriage experiences (either in the form of calling a doctor to the house or through visiting a hospital). Further, families also had to hand over the tissues, or as discussed earlier, doctors could mislead their patients in order to remove tissues from the home. But we cannot forget the power that women, their families, and their attendants held over the initial step of turning a fetus into a specimen.

For those doctors who were successful, once they removed fetal and placental tissues from patients' homes, they could then introduce them into more well-established scientific locations, such as professional meetings, university classrooms, and museums. Often, doctors sought to share these materials with a larger group, with the most popular audience being the medical society. On the evening of August 7, 1855, a Dr. White arrived at the Buffalo Medical Association with a human ovum to share with the group. He recounted that a patient, believing herself pregnant for the fourth time, called in medical aid when she suffered abdominal pains. Three months later, after a string of remedies and treatments, she passed the ovum. White claimed that "it had thus been retained three and a half months after death, and was a good illustration of . . . the antiseptic qualities" of the amniotic fluid. Discussion followed, in which physicians speculated on why this fetus was in such good condition when other specimens that remained in the uterus long after their death emerged in a more decayed state. Dr. White concluded the discussion with the point that "there was, perhaps, room for question as to whether the death of the foetus depended on the mother, or vice versa."[67] This well-preserved fetus called into question the very nature of the physical relationship between mother and fetus.

Over the next few decades, the medical periodicals were peppered with similar reports from meetings across the country. In 1857, a Dr. Coale presented a seven-month fetus before the Boston Society for Medical Improvement; ten years later, a Dr. Markoe exhibited a four-month fetus for the New York Pathological Society; in 1873, Dr. J. V. Ingham presented, on behalf of a colleague, an ovum in the eighth week of gestation at the Philadelphia Obstetrical Society; in 1878, Dr. Achilles presented to the Evansville Medical Society a "much flattened" fetus of four and a half months; J. H. Etheridge brought a three-month fetus to the Chicago Gynecological Society in 1885; and in 1888, Dr. E. P. Murdock brought a three-month fetus to the Chicago Pathological Society.[68] In 1871, a Dr. Warner exhibited a diseased fetus, "of some four and a half months," before the Gynaecological Society of Boston, sparking such interest that the president of the society appointed a committee to "make a microscopal examination of the specimen, which was different from anything that had been seen by any of the members."[69]

Physicians not only displayed and discussed fetal specimens at medical society meetings, but they also relocated the tissues to universities and hospitals and integrated them into medical education. After attending a six-months pregnant woman experiencing "grinding and benumbing pains," P. Claiborne Gooch walked away with a fetus that he then gave to his friend Professor C. P. Johnson to exhibit to the class of the Richmond Medical College in 1852.[70] Theophilus Parvin opened one of his lectures of clinical obstetrics at the Philadelphia Hospital by declaring, "I show you here a fetus with cord and placenta, the fetus having been dead some days before its expulsion, as is proved by its presenting the condition known as maceration, which will be spoken of in a few minutes."[71] Other physicians included references to the appearance of miscarried fetuses within the pages of their teaching textbooks.[72] For most doctors, transforming the fetal tissues into specimens required separating them from their domestic origins (a woman's bed, bedroom, house, or arms) and introducing them in physical locations that both doctors and the public would recognize as scientific.

The second form of scientific integration came in the presentation of these tissues, how physicians not only physically separated the miscarriage materials from their female patients who delivered them, but then also presented the tissues as something completely removed from women, pregnancy, and family. Throughout the latter half of the nineteenth century, American doctors refashioned fetal tissues into specimens by illustratively depicting them as independent beings, and by physically placing them in jars. Both of these methods further entangled the tiny creatures into a world of science while simultaneously further disentangling them from a family or a mother.

When Alex Garnett, the Washington, D.C., physician who bemoaned a family's refusal to his request to take a five-month-old fetus away after a case of miscarriage, could not physically investigate "the specimen" further in his office with a microscope, he instead made a drawing of the fetus at his patient's home and included the illustration in his write-up of the case that appeared in the *American Journal of the Medical Sciences* in 1880. In his seven-page article (quite lengthy by the era's standards), Garnett detailed the appearance of the fetus, including how the umbilical cord, while "apparently healthy, [and] of usual length" was wrapped twice around the body and abnormally fused with the placenta. Garnett then included his drawing, which shows a small, childlike figure, curled up and shrouded in the shaded bubble of the placenta. The aspect of the drawing Garnett depicted as important, the fusion of the umbilical cord and the placenta, is too shaded to clearly see; instead, the viewer is drawn to the large, bowed head of the fetus and its small pointed nose. Nowhere in the text or the image does Garnett refer to where this creature would naturally be housed—in a woman's body. Instead, we are confronted with a floating, independent being, one created not by a reproducing woman in a domestic setting, but one created by a medical professional in the pages of a scientific journal.[73]

Doctors also relied on physically presenting fetal specimens primarily in jars, which were often filled with alcohol for preservation (formaldehyde was not widely commercially available until around 1900). While the jar may seem like a practical solution to the problem of how to carry around a small fleshy object while hopefully preventing it from rotting, this container also signified

Fig. 1.

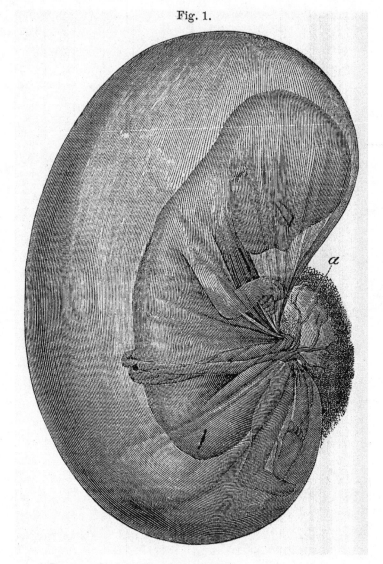

FIG. 8. Drawing included in Alex Garnett's article in the *American Journal of the Medical Sciences* (1880). (Ebling Library's Rare Books and Special Collections, University of Wisconsin–Madison)

the growing importance of scientific markers in American medicine, and it stood in stark contrast to an alternative possible presentation—a coffin or urn. An important aspect of Dr. Lopez's saga in bringing a fetus from a case of miscarriage to a medical meeting was the breaking of the jar of alcohol. Lopez chose a container that could halt the natural process of degradation while also allowing others to see this valuable creature he carried with him.

In his 1882 professional advice manual, *The Physician Himself and What He Should Add to the Strictly Scientific*, physician D. W. Cathell recommended that a physician should display mementos of his dissections and pathological and anatomical specimens in his office, alongside the requisite skeleton, microscope, and diplomas.[74] Such specimens undoubtedly should be kept in glass jars of alcohol, so that potential patients could see the scientific nature of the physician's skill and marvel at how he was able to reveal the hidden mysteries of the human body. As the nineteenth century progressed, the place of science gained new respect in the everyday practice of the regular physician, and jars filled with specimens, including fetal specimens, could be markers of a doctor's scientific knowledge and skill.

In 1896, Dr. William Stevens published his account of a miscarriage utilizing both means of presentation, crafting the tissues he gained in practice as purely scientific with no seeming connection to domestic reproduction. Stevens presented four specimens to the Michigan State Medical Society to illustrate his thoughts on partial abortion; each specimen was neatly floating in a glass jar of alcohol, and the journal *Transactions of the Michigan State Medical Society* later printed a photograph of them. Unlike Garnett's illustration, Stevens's specimens bore no resemblance to children, and instead more resembled a gallstone or tumor. The neat jars nestled in his professional publication easily signal the specimens as scientific objects with no connection to childbirth, mothering, or kinship.[75]

In December 1867, Dr. George Hopkins was called in to see a Mrs. M. for the birth of her child. Once he successfully delivered the infant and placenta, Hopkins examined the woman's uterus and

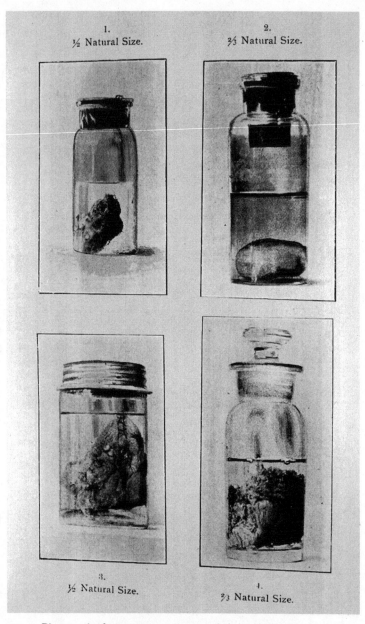

1.
½ Natural Size.

2.
⅔ Natural Size.

3.
½ Natural Size.

4.
⅔ Natural Size.

FIG. 9. Photograph of miscarriage specimens included in William Stevens's article in *Transactions of the Michigan State Medical Society* (1896). (Ebling Library's Rare Books and Special Collections, University of Wisconsin–Madison)

found a "mass about the size of a hen's egg." Hopkins removed it and because it seemed peculiar in appearance, he saved it for further study. Once he concluded the case, Hopkins took the mass back to his office, where he sectioned it, and put it under the microscope and determined it to be a degenerated ovum about three months in age.[76]

In 1887, Dr. Julia Carpenter attended to a Mrs. B., who had miscarried her previous pregnancy and was bleeding in the second month of her latest one. Carpenter, who believed the first miscarriage was the result of "one of the greatest drains of all the reserve forces of the body, two years of uninterrupted gay society life," quickly deemed another miscarriage inevitable. Mrs. B. delivered a small ovum, clearly younger than two months, and Carpenter informed her patient that another ovum could still remain, which she subsequently delivered some weeks later. In the case of the first ovum, Carpenter shared it with Dr. Thaddeus Reamy, and together they determined it to be the age of three weeks, and she wrote: "it was about an inch in length and, as it was floated in water, the fringe-like villi of the chorion showed beautifully." In the case of the second mass, Carpenter took the tissues to the office of Dr. Reamy, "where it was dissected, and pronounced to be a product of conception."[77]

For Carpenter and Hopkins, and many other nineteenth-century physicians, dissecting, floating, and analyzing fetal tissues under a microscope helped to recraft the materials of miscarriage into specimens. While Hopkins departed the house of his female patient with a full-term baby left behind, completely entangled in its new family, he took along with him an ovum, which required further work to integrate instead into a world of science and research. Hopkins took the tissues to his medical office, where he sectioned it and completed the transfer from family to specimen by publishing his results in a medical journal. Likewise, Carpenter easily carried two ova out of a patient's home, shared them with a colleague, floated one, dissected the other, and published commentary on both.

Often physicians like Hopkins and Carpenter would carry out all three steps of incorporating miscarriage materials into the world of medical science, showing how the methods could work together seamlessly. However, I think this scientific integration work is revealed more clearly when physicians were restricted from carrying out all three steps and were left to incorporate these specimens into science where they could. For example, let us return to the case of Dr. Charles Munde and his wife who miscarried in 1850. The Mundes had just arrived from Europe, and Dr. Munde had yet to form professional alliances or even learn where the local medical society met, so he was left with retaining the miscarriage products in his home. However, as he described it, he placed the tissues in a jar of alcohol. In this liminal space of both medical encounter and perhaps personal disappointment, Munde still undertook to transform the products into a preserved specimen, as well as write up his observations for publication.

This transformation of miscarriage products into fetal specimens did not remain internal to medical writings or behind the closed doors of medical society meetings, but rather, it became an accepted image of the fetus in public as well. In fact, if we look beyond the medical literature, we can see how successful, or perhaps how necessary, these reentanglements were for more public approval of the emerging medical and scientific interest in human fetuses. Magazine and newspaper stories from the late nineteenth century reveal how some nonscientists viewed the fetus and its place in society.

In 1898, Joanna R. Nicholls Kyle wrote a report for the popular publication *Godey's Magazine* on a visit to the Army Medical Library and Museum in Washington, D.C. In what would turn out to be the last year of the long-running and popular women's magazine (previously known as *Godey's Lady Book*), Kyle described visiting the new public museum, which housed thousands of human specimens. The Army Medical Museum got its start during the Civil War, when then U.S. Surgeon General William Hammond directed all Union doctors to collect examples of "morbid anatomy" and ship them to his office in D. C. for cataloging, future research, and placement alongside the library he was also building. Collection of body parts, organs, skin sections, and photographs of a wide variety of injuries and diseases continued after the war, and by the 1880s the collection had overgrown its housing, prompting the federal government to build a new home for the books and specimens, which was completed in 1887. In the intervening years, the anatomical collection had grown beyond the amputated limbs and bullet-ridden organs of the war to include any human specimen deemed worthy of study by the larger American medical community.[78]

Kyle visited the museum (on the second floor of the new building; the remaining floors served as laboratories and other research spaces) in 1898 and filed a detailed report on the history of the museum and library, its current collection, and its role as a tourist attraction. According to Kyle, the collection held over 33,000 specimens, including gunshot wounds, a wide variety of bones, skin diseases, sections of frozen bodies, drawings of parasites, wax models of sperm and egg, and a large collection of human fetuses and embryos in jars. Keeping her popular audience in mind, Kyle reported on particular objects of interest, such as "a bit of human skin on which an arrow had been tattooed."

In the Army Medical Museum's first decade, tens of thousands visited each year to see the array of specimens.[79] It is significant that Joanna Kyle, while describing the examples of skin conditions as "revolting" and the displays of the ravages of disease as "hideous," used the term "delicate" when discussing some of the embryological preparations. In the closing of her article, Kyle promoted the value of the museum for public edification. She also encouraged her readers to think of the museum for public school class visits and as a fine outing for families with young children.[80] The fetuses on display there, framed within glass and mounted in the physical location of a museum, garnered no outrage or criticism, but instead they seemed to Kyle to fit perfectly within the larger world of research and science.

Public fetuses unmoored from scientific entanglements were interpreted quite differently. A *New York Times* article from

1877 brings us the story of Mrs. Mary Tait and her miscarriage. Mrs. Tait was rushed to the New York Hospital after receiving two stab wounds in her abdomen. Five days later, she delivered a six-month-old fetus and returned home soon after. The hospital morgue received a burial permit for the fetus and sent Dan Russel, the driver of the dead wagon, to collect. When Russel arrived, "he was told by the clerk that he guessed the body had been thrown into the furnace and cremated. Dan's astonishment and horror at the supposed barbarity of the physicians knew no bounds." When a *Times* reporter interviewed physicians at the hospital, one stated that he didn't understand the protests, and he actually "seemed greatly amused at the interest created by the occurrence." Another stated that if the fetus had been cremated, "he could see nothing improper in it. He did not know whether such a proceeding was common in hospitals, but it was common to burn parts of limbs that had been amputated." It was, after all, the doctor reported, the most effective method of disposal.[81]

Other newspapers described fetuses that were found distinctly outside of science as criminal, if not abhorrent. In 1895, two boys fishing in the Missouri River in Sioux City, Iowa, discovered a human fetus, floating along, wrapped in a bed quilt.[82] In 1898, a human fetus was discovered in the hills around Los Angeles.[83] In both cases, police quickly became involved, and even though the authorities could not determine how the fetuses arrived in the river or the hills, each case was depicted as a deplorable crime.

When a fetus became detached from its entanglements either of family or of scientific research, as with these cases, words such as "barbarity" were bandied about in the press. In the *New York Times* article, the fetus was located not in a bedroom or a lecture hall, but in a hospital furnace, a location typically reserved for amputated body parts or other waste. This fetus was located in a liminal space between child and specimen, and between person and depersonalized body. Whereas at the Army Medical Museum, where fetuses resided in a scientific building, in jars of alcohol, and displayed for the betterment of scientific knowledge, the specimens garnered no outcry or scandal that I have been able to find.

Conclusion

Miscarriage accounts in nineteenth-century medical literature shed light on a rather unique collecting practice, as obtaining a human fetus or embryo was fundamentally different from acquiring other kinds of embryological specimens. Obtaining human specimens was not as simple as scooping up fish embryos from the stream in the backyard, or cracking open an egg; in the nineteenth century, miscarrying women were the primary source of embryological specimens. Women, along with their families, played a pivotal role in determining the nature of the tissues coming from their bodies (fetus, clot, child), and what should be done with them. This history of miscarriage brings us keen insight into the messy world of early embryology—a field that involved family tragedies, personal joy, and bodies in jars.

Furthermore, examining doctors' interest in fetal tissues and their actions to refashion them into scientific specimens allows us a new view into the roots of our own contemporary science and politics of reproduction. Lennart Nilsson's iconic images of fetal development in a 1965 issue of *Life* magazine stand as a modern example of the situational construction of fetal tissues. Nilsson's pictures, including the cover image of an eighteen-week-old fetus posed as a sleeping child, are often used to exemplify the "scientific" proof of the humanization of an early fetus.[84] However, had *Life* magazine shown that very same fetus (most likely the result of an abortion or miscarriage) instead in a trash bag or carelessly thrown on a hillside, the resulting reaction would probably have been extremely negative. Today fetal tissues are used for a number of scientific research projects investigating a range of diseases and treatments, without much public scrutiny. However, when they are disentangled from this world of pure science, such as in the case of abortion providers supposedly profiting from the sale of fetal bodies and parts, suddenly we see discussions of the "barbarity" of those involved.

In the second half of the nineteenth century American physicians recognized the significance of miscarriage products as snapshots of human development. And while the collection of these snap-shots required a large host of participants, each creating their own meaning of the fetus along the way, the work carried out by physicians to entangle these fetal bodies in networks of science remains with us today. As we encounter legal debates about fetal person-hood, fetal pain, and fetal rights, we cannot forget that much of the "evidence" in these debates rests on the creation and construction of the American fetus as a scientific specimen.

One of the major conceptual shifts for nineteenth-century physicians was in how they interpreted miscarriage and the result-ing tissues in terms of "normal." As discussed earlier, until around the 1830s, most doctors agreed that the results of miscarriage were examples of abnormal development—fruit, gristle, or moles, but not normal humans. By the 1880s, doctors instead were deeply involved in referring to miscarriage products as examples of normal human development, even while they were also describing miscarriage as abnormal. This may seem contradictory, and I think it is. If doctors claimed that miscarriage was an abnormal end to pregnancy, then how could they also claim that specimens collected from miscar-riage illustrated normal development and provided insights into normal human physiology and death? This unacknowledged con-tradiction reveals how much doctors valued miscarriage products as scientific specimens. Because medical researchers viewed these tissues as being so rich in information that was impossible to gain any other way, they were willing to overlook the contradiction of normality.

By the 1870s, many American women had the opportunity to see human fetuses through diagrams, drawings, and models. Popu-lar health books presented images of fertilized eggs, early embryo-logical divisions, and the fetus that could be discernable as early as the second month of gestation.[85] The new science of embryology also appeared in public forums. In addition to the large collection on display at the Army Medical Museum, a display of embryo-logical wax models, measuring eight feet high and almost fifteen feet wide and comprised of human and animal specimens, was exhibited at the World's Fair in Chicago in 1893; this presentation of the bodies housed by pregnancy attracted thousands daily.[86]

It is within this context that we can better understand why families would so freely hand over miscarriage materials—some women were relieved, or even overjoyed, at the event of miscarriage, and for those who were less than thrilled about being pregnant, seeing the lost pregnancy as a specimen may have been emotionally helpful.[87] Remembering the relief of Emily FitzGerald ("I am thankful now that I did have it"), the contentment of Annie Van Ness ("I am happy again"), and the pleasure of Mary Cheney ("O Bliss, O Rapture unforeseen!") over their miscarriages helps to explain the relative ease of medical access to fetal tissues. For the many women who could not gain access to contraception or abortion (or could not coincide either with their personal beliefs), thinking of miscarriage as "flooding" or the passage of clots or specimens afforded some recourse to constant reproduction and childcare. In an era of little reproductive control or even low expectation of success for each pregnancy, women and doctors could easily consider a human fetus as a specimen or "a jointed doll." In the end, the history of miscarriage reveals the many actors—doctors, scientists, and reproducing women—who worked together and fashioned a world that reshaped blood and clots into valuable research objects and representations of the wonder of mankind.

Conclusion

In September 2009, Penelope Trunk, a blogger and entrepreneur, posted to her Twitter feed: "I'm in a board meeting. Having a miscarriage. Thank goodness, because there's a fucked-up 3-week hoop-jump to have an abortion in Wisconsin."[1] Her post garnered a slew of press where journalists lambasted her for "TMI" and ABC News interviewed a clinical psychologist who doubted Trunk could truly be as callous as she appeared: "I think there's more ambivalence she's not acknowledging."[2] Her blog received hundreds of comments, most of them negative, including one that stated: "To tweet about something that devastates other women you found relief. You are a poor excuse for a human being."[3]

When Trunk appeared on CNN to respond to some of her critics, anchorman Rick Sanchez asked her, "Have you no shame?" and censured her for "treating the birth of a human being so casually." Throughout the interview, Trunk cited the statistic that 75 percent of all women have a miscarriage and claimed, "it's a natural part of women being women."[4] In an article written for the *Guardian*, Trunk considered the outcry her post created and reported, "I am not sure why people think there is a 'correct' emotion for miscarriage. For anything, really."[5]

While many people found Trunk's post disturbing, they were not united in their reasons. Some claimed that she should not have provided such intimate details in a public forum, while others found her discussion of this bodily function disgusting or offensive. Still others (on both sides of the abortion debate) found her treatment of miscarriage cold and insensitive. Trunk attempted to use the publicity to criticize Wisconsin abortion laws, but most of the press focused instead on her publicizing what was considered by many to be a private matter. Trunk was skewered in the press and on social media in effect for breaking the silence around miscarriage.

In the summer of 2015, Facebook founder Mark Zuckerberg announced the pregnancy of his wife, Priscilla Chan, and he included in the announcement (via Facebook, of course) the news that the couple had been trying to have children for many years and had suffered three miscarriages along the way. Zuckerberg described their miscarriage experiences as lonely and supposed that most people did not discuss miscarriage because "you worry your problems will distance you or reflect upon you—as if you're defective or did something to cause this." Unlike Trunk's tweet, Zuckerberg's disclosure received thousands of positive comments.[6] Of course, Zuckerberg did not express relief over his wife's miscarriages; he painted them as struggles along the way to the intended goal: a healthy baby. While we may be in a new age of miscarriage openness, so far the most appropriate miscarriage discussion is one that revolves around loss, sadness, and grief. Women like Trunk, who might feel ambivalent or even relief at a miscarriage, may still be criticized, perpetrating the silence around pregnancy loss.

This study has described the many complicated factors involved in a woman's interpretation of miscarriage. In nineteenth-century America those factors included family size, financial concerns, geographic environment, personal desires, and religious beliefs. A century and a half later, although we might have different reproductive agendas, gender roles, and economic frameworks, we share many of these concerns, even if we are told not to talk about them or told that there is an expected and correct response. Women still have pregnancies that they want, ones that they dread, and ones about which they feel uncertain.

Perhaps most importantly, this project has uncovered personal stories of women who struggled with pregnancy and pregnancy loss in nineteenth-century America. These tales, which have remained hidden for so long, reveal the experience of reproducing in the past. Examining the experiences of a woman struggling for survival in the Alaskan frontier alongside those of a woman living in the lap of luxury in Europe allow us to get closer to understanding what it meant to be pregnant in the nineteenth century, and what it meant to watch and feel that pregnancy slip away. The picture that results is one of American women struggling to control their fertility and their lives. Many nineteenth-century women expressed pregnancy loss in terms of ill fortune, God's plan, or other forces beyond their control. When wanting to limit their family's size or control their reproductive status but having little in the way to make that happen, some women could only interpret miscarriage in a more benign manner.

While this book describes the complex forces that shaped a woman's response to miscarriage in the nineteenth century, it also challenges the notion that pregnancy loss can or should carry any innate meaning. Although numerous groups in today's society support the idea that the "correct" and somehow inherent understanding of miscarriage is the tragic death of a baby, this understanding leaves many women feeling isolated and uncomfortable. Some readers may find a personal connection with the disappointment and sorrow expressed by Lucretia Everett, but there are others who would equally identify with Mary Cheney's and Annie Van Ness's effusions of joy at the loss of their pregnancies.

By revealing the connections between pregnancy loss and death, embryology, professionalization, and illness, this study illuminates the multifaceted nature of miscarriage. The loss of a pregnancy in the nineteenth century was a changing and changeable construct. In an era without effective or legal means of fertility control and when many Americans found little certainty that every pregnancy could or should result in a live, healthy birth, the interpretations of miscarriage were shaped by individuals in accordance with their desires, fears, and daily lives.

In our current medically shaped reproductive world, each pregnancy includes a fetus and, to some, a child from the very beginning. But these constructs are shaped by a woman's ability to exercise control over her fertility. Despite the realities many American women face, which can include lost pregnancies, fertility struggles, or lack of access to contraception, pregnancy is commonly depicted as an easy, purposeful, and wanted condition. While feminist scholars celebrate the triumphs of the wider availability of fertility control gained over the last century, we need to also acknowledge the potential losses incurred by this achievement. The prevailing assumption that all women retain control over their own fertility has resulted in a universal image of pregnancy as wanted, protected, monitored, celebrated, and always resulting in a healthy baby. This universal understanding of pregnancy leaves little room for women who have felt conflicted about their own pregnancies, faced reproductive-control restrictions, or lost their pregnancies or newborns. The individuality and fluidity of pregnancy interpretations revealed by nineteenth-century personal writings has perhaps been an unintended victim of the success of the birth control movement. Women may feel able to better control how many children to have and when, but perhaps they also feel particularly responsible when they have difficulty achieving or sustaining pregnancy. In addition, women with unwanted pregnancies or women who feel ambiguous about their pregnant bodies may find themselves marginalized in our culture of fertility confidence and value.[7]

Miscarriage, then and now, occupies a provocative liminal space in multiple regards. It is primarily understood as a natural bodily event, and yet the abnormal end to a pregnancy. It is not really a death and yet not quite a birth. It may not produce a child or a mother, but it remains an important aspect of mothering and childbearing. Situated in this space, miscarriage is perfectly oriented to reveal deeper meanings of the categories involved: mother, child, pregnant, normal, and natural. Miscarriage thus serves as a valuable cultural signifier, and rather than marginalize discussions about it, we should bring it into our conversations about gender, bodies, families, and identity.

This project opens the door to a variety of future studies in both women's history and medical history. It is easy to assume a link exists between miscarriage and motherhood. Yet, as the history of miscarriage demonstrates, the nineteenth-century pregnant body was not necessarily a maternal body. Lucretia Everett, who experienced many miscarriages but never a live birth, did not consider herself a mother. Neither women nor doctors considered pregnancy loss as a maternal failing, suggesting that motherhood began only at birth. As many nineteenth-century Americans would not have considered the fetus a child, they also did not consider pregnancy as making a mother. However, scholars have shown that a woman could become a maternal body through other pathways, such as adoption or through social avenues to mothering like the child-raising duties of nursemaids or enslaved women put in the role of "mammy."[8] These studies together indicate that the construct of the maternal body was and is a complex process that involves social, racial, and corporeal aspects.

This study also points to the importance of developments in the early and mid-twentieth century in the formation of our modern understanding of the human fetus and pregnancy. In the previous century, women felt they had little control over the fates of their pregnancies, and doctors invested little energy in policing the behavior of pregnant women. I suspect that further research into pregnancy in the first half of the twentieth century would illuminate how both women and doctors assisted in the creation of notions of the modern fetus and the modern pregnancy.[9] With the developments in prenatal health care, improved birth control, decreasing infant mortality, and shifts in gender roles and family constructs, did women begin to understand their pregnancies differently? Further research could unveil the extent to which women played an active and important role in the establishment of their own position as protectors of fetal life.

This history of miscarriage also opens doors in the study of interactions among doctors, scientists, and women in the realm of embryology. By unveiling the embryological interests and work of American physicians, this study begins to address previously neglected sources in the history of biology. However, more work can and should be done to connect these medical endeavors to the work of American biologists in the nineteenth century. While many scientists undoubtedly discounted the embryological work of doctors, there was still an important link between the two groups via the tissues they shared. American biologists were dependent on doctors for fetal tissues, and how did this association shape early embryology? Both doctors and scientists were also ultimately dependent on women for the donation of fetal tissues, and an exploration into this tissue trade could reveal fascinating insights into the very meaning of human. Early understandings of the human fetus and how it developed were shaped in many stages, by the women who offered up tissues and declared them normal, by the doctors who received these tissues and further judged the normality of them, and finally by biologists, who attempted to place these tissues into a scientific discourse. While my study only begins to make headway into understanding these relationships, it uncovers the existence of such tissue movements, and I hope it will prompt others to inquire into these complex trade networks.

Finally, this examination of nineteenth-century miscarriage both supports and calls into question the accepted wisdom that our current sense of maternal guilt in cases of miscarriage should be placed squarely on the shoulders of technology and the women's health movement. A common narrative claims that our modern inclination to personify the fetus is solely linked to our ability to see it in all its human detail.[10] Women and doctors in the nineteenth century did not view pregnancy as inclusive of another person, and hence there was little agreement on requiring women to protect those "people" or blaming mothers when pregnancies failed. These findings support that idea that such understandings of pregnancy and pregnancy loss developed later in the twentieth century.

However, the claim that visualization technologies, such as ultrasound, were one of the major drivers of the momentous shift in conceptions of pregnancy becomes muddied when we examine the nineteenth century. Many women encountered visual and physical models of the developing human fetus in the nineteenth century. I would argue that the ultrasound image of one's own child carries vast qualitative differences from the wax model of a standard embryo, but I still think this dissemination of the image of embryos in the nineteenth century calls into question the simplicity of the argument that women began to believe in the idea that pregnancy included another person only when they were shown what that person looked like. Instead, this study indicates that this transition in reproductive thinking was much more complex. Were women more interested in looking at their fetuses and creating new identities for them once other factors had fallen into place, such as effective birth control, lower infant mortality, and legalized abortion? While women remained in a world where they had little and often no control over their fertility, they might be more apt to see their miscarriages as being subject to fortune and fate, and less interested in thinking of their pregnant bellies as holding another person. But once pregnancy became more controllable and its fate more predictable, women could begin to think of a person within.

How women described their pregnant and miscarrying bodies, or how they expressed their reproductive struggles and joys reveals more than narratives of pregnancy loss. The close readings of the experiences of Abigail Adams, Lucretia Everett, Mary Longfellow, Rachel Cormany, Alice Bodman, Elizabeth Cabot, Emily FitzGerald, Ellen Garrison, Katherine Norton, Dolly Burge, Gertrude Thomas, Susan Magoffin, Caroline Dall, Annie Van Ness, Mary Cheney, and Blanche Ames offer us insights into how these women negotiated the social, cultural, economic, political, racial, and medical landscape in their time and worked to create families, identities, and communities. Through these individual stories we can better understand how a wealthy woman might feel joy at a miscarriage, how a young bride would become unhappy about her pregnancy, and how Mrs. T.J.B. could hand over a four-month-old fetus to her physician so that he could study it further and share it with his colleagues.

Historical value aside, personal stories of modern pregnancy loss can help us better understand the cultural silence around it and begin to break it apart. Only when we consider why women keep silent about their miscarriages, and all the various and complex reasons, can we have any hope of compelling them, their doctors, their families, and everyone to speak out about miscarriage. While some women undoubtedly have no interest in publicly sharing their stories of miscarriage, we need to work toward creating a safe space for women who do want to share. Only through speaking out and examining how miscarriage works in individual lives can we make progress in combating the deleterious mental, emotional, and physical effects of the experience.

Maggie was thirty-eight and had two children when she had her third miscarriage.[11] She had been through the experience before and knew what to expect in terms of bleeding and pain. When she first became pregnant this time, Maggie was openly ambivalent about the pregnancy, and she had told friends and family: "I thought I was done with babies." When she lost the pregnancy, she was more occupied with how to break the news to her children than about any grief she might have been feeling. When she visited her midwife afterwards, she was surprised to find the woman outraged at Maggie's lack of visible grief. The midwife reprimanded Maggie for not feeling sad, for not caring enough about the pregnancy. After the exchange, Maggie told very few people about the miscarriage.

Anna was thirty-seven when she had her second miscarriage. Also taken by surprise by the pregnancy, Anna was unsure how she felt about it. She and her husband had been discussing the possibility of having more children ever since the birth of their second child five years earlier, but they had not decided one way or the other. But now, Anna had just started a new job, had earned only two sick days, and did not want her employers to think she had deceived them into hiring someone who would immediately need parental leave. She used both sick days to take care of the miscarriage (it started on one day, but she could not get an appointment for a D&C until the next day) and told coworkers it was the flu.

I was thirty-five when I had my first miscarriage. My partner and I had been trying to get pregnant for over a year, and I was ecstatic when I saw the blue lines on the pregnancy test. Only a few weeks later, I started to bleed and instantly knew what was happening (one of the benefits of studying miscarriage for the past decade).

Later, after sitting in the emergency room for hours, it struck me that not once had a nurse, doctor, technician, or administrative staff member who saw me used the word "miscarriage." I was told that they could not find my "pregnancy" on the ultrasound, that I might have lost "the pregnancy," and I was discharged with the diagnosis "incomplete abortion." I had a lunch meeting scheduled that day with the chair of my department. I sent him an email from the hospital, citing a "medical issue," worried that telling him I was having a miscarriage might make him uncomfortable.

These three individual stories reveal just three of the multitude of reasons why women stay silent about their miscarriages. We worry about how others will judge our reactions, we worry what the phenomenon might mean about us as employees (in a world where most women still have male supervisors and little paid leave), and we worry that because it is not a common topic of conversation our story might make others uncomfortable. And in a twist that I did not see coming when I started this project, we learn this silence from our medical system. I left the hospital wondering if I had even been pregnant, if I had lost something, if I could even truthfully say that I had had a miscarriage. If the medical "experts" I had consulted did not tell me I had a miscarriage, then perhaps I didn't.

In recent years, the medical community has begun to study the silence surrounding miscarriage and how that might impact women and their partners. In 2015, a team of researchers conducted a national survey and found that 47 percent of respondents who had experienced miscarriage felt guilty, 41 percent reported thinking they had done something wrong, 41 percent felt alone, and 28 percent felt ashamed. The article in *Obstetrics and Gynecology* presenting results from this survey argues that this culture of silence harms women by helping to cause this guilt and shame, but the researchers do not explore their own role in perpetrating this silence.[12] How are women to feel comfortable speaking out about their miscarriages if their doctors, acknowledged by many in our current culture to be the experts on the topic, do not use the term? Medical language and categories cannot be separated from social constructs, and thus part of the change to put a stop to this damaging silence needs to come from the medical community.

To fully understand how we got to where we are today—the shame, the loneliness, the silence—we need to consider the reproductive freedoms gained over the course of the last hundred years, those gains that historians usually write about only in terms of triumph and progress. Annie Van Ness and her compatriots did not have access to effective birth control, could not easily or legally obtain an abortion, and were often misadvised about when their "safe" days for sex were. As contraception and abortion became legal, safe, effective, and affordable for more American women in the latter half of the twentieth century, and as scientists untangled the physiology of pregnancy to better understand how it happens and how to avoid it, many women came to feel that they had absolute control over when they got pregnant. That sense of control only increased with advances in artificial insemination, leading many Americans to believe that modern medicine can fix any reproductive problem. But with great control always comes great responsibility. Because women do have such unprecedented control over their fertility, how many now feel that, when something goes wrong, it must be their fault? Perhaps we can start to learn from women like Mary Cheney and embrace instead a variety of miscarriage interpretations, emotions, and realities.

Acknowledgments

It is my great pleasure to thank all of those who helped build, nurture, and sustain this book over the past ten years. This project began as a doctoral dissertation at the University of Wisconsin–Madison, and I am endlessly thankful to my advisor, Judith Houck, for helping me discover my voice and continuing to push me academically while providing warm support. The academic community in the Department of History of Science, Medicine, and Technology at UW provided a welcoming home to begin my career; my colleagues, teachers, and friends there continue to shape my work and help me find balance.

I am grateful for the financial support I received for this project at multiple stages. A Bain Scholar-in-Residence Fellowship from Smith College and a Countway Library Fellowship in the History of Medicine from Harvard University enabled me to discover key primary sources tracing individual women's stories through diaries, letters, physicians' reports, and hospital records. The Department of the History of Science, Medicine, and Technology at UW awarded me a William Coleman Dissertation Fellowship and a Maurice L. Richardson Fellowship, which granted me productive time to finish my dissertation and begin reshaping it into a monograph. The two years I spent as an ACLS New Faculty Fellow at Duke University were crucial for providing additional research and writing time.

Librarians and archivists across the country proved invaluable to the success of this project. The staff at both the Sophia Smith Collection and the Countway Library showed enthusiasm for my work and dug out beautiful images and key documents. Collections at the Massachusetts Historical Society, the Schlesinger Library at Radcliffe College, and the Wisconsin Historical Society contained important sources for contextual details for many of the women profiled here. A few librarians deserve special mention. Micaela Sullivan-Fowler at the Ebling Library at UW is the kind of librarian that all researchers love. From the first time she allowed me into the secret cage of old volumes to the final weeks of this book manuscript when she generously shared images of floating fetuses, she has constantly amazed me and enriched my scholarship. Rachel Ingold at the Rubenstein Library at Duke will forever be in my debt for introducing me to Charles Brayton and for her continued support years after my short stay in Durham.

My department at the University of New Mexico has shown incredible support from the very beginning. When Durwood Ball walked up to me after my job talk and handed me Susan Shelby Magoffin's letters, with her description of her miscarriage marked, I knew I was in a good place. My fellow historians have shown tremendous encouragement and assistance with my scholarship and my family. Special thanks to Cathleen Cahill, Luis Campos, Sarah and Jon Davis-Secord, Tiffany Florvil, David Prior, Brian Goldstein, Theresa McCulla, and Virginia Scharff for drinks, laughs, and sanity.

Numerous scholars have provided constructive feedback on this project. Portions of this work have appeared in national conferences, including multiple meetings of the American Association of the History of Medicine, the History of Science Society meeting, and the Berkshire Conference of Women Historians. Each time, my fellow historians have provided valuable comments and helped sustain my enthusiasm for the project. At Rutgers University Press, I am particularly grateful to the two readers of my manuscript, Leslie Reagan and Lara Freidenfelds. Their thorough comments and suggestions challenged me and improved the book considerably. No stranger to this project, Lara has been an important champion of my work since we organized a conference panel on miscarriage back in 2008. Peter Mickulas has been a fantastic editor and a pleasure to work with.

I cannot thank enough those friends who encouraged me and helped cultivate my curiosity and drive throughout the long process. Two decades ago, Jade Huang, Sun Kim, Sally McGrane, and Meghan Sullivan helped me realize I liked history and wanted to read about it all the time, and our times in San Francisco, Baltimore, and D.C. will forever remain happy and important memories. Erika Milam, a wonderful mentor to a first-year grad student, is still the most insightful and kind scholar I know. The wonderful friends I made in graduate school, Andrew Ruis, Theresa Pesavento, Jesse and Claire Taylor, Judy and Howard Kaplan, Kellen Backer, and Annie Rauh, have given me professional and personal support at various points in my scholarly career, and I would not have survived the process in any happy way without them. Cathy and Gerard Leahy provided invaluable contributions to the book through babysitting, brewery exploring, and many inappropriate music nights.

My mother was the first person to show me how fascinating the lives of common people, especially women, in the past could be, and all of my historical work is rooted in her enthusiasm. My father supported each of my new career paths without question and kept his pride in my accomplishments constant. Megan, Heather, and Amber: I would be insane, adrift, and depressed without you in my life. My scholarship is ever improving because you always have my back. As I write these lines, my son is yelling from another room about what he has put in the potty, reminding me of all the academic mamas who can never be one without the other. Like all of you women juggling work and motherhood, I survive only because of those who help hold me up. Fred Gibbs has done most of that holding, making countless meals, occupying a toddler through numerous conferences, and editing thousands of pages with little complaint. He has helped me through every stage of this book, and his love and support for both Miles and me makes this world, miscarriages and all, a happier place.

Notes

Introduction

1. Clara Crowninshield, *Diary: A European Tour with Longfellow, 1835–1836*, ed. Andrew R. Hilen (Seattle: University of Washington Press, 1956), 136.
2. Ibid., note 10.
3. Ibid., 158.
4. For examples of the language used to describe miscarriage in two of the more widely read sources for popular reproductive knowledge, see the websites for *What to Expect When You're Expecting*, http://www.whattoexpect.com/pregnancy/emotional-life/grief-and-loss/coping-with-a-miscarriage.aspx; and *Our Bodies Ourselves*, http://www.ourbodiesourselves.org/book/childbirthexcerpt.asp?id=80. Both last accessed June 6, 2017.
5. This book is based on five major sets of sources: medical teaching texts, medical periodical literature, domestic health guides, women's personal writings, and hospital records, all from 1820 to 1912. The published medical literature focuses on American editions or publications, although for the early nineteenth century I did rely on medical texts originally published in Europe, but I limited myself to those discussed widely in American medical journals. In the end, this book is based on a survey of over two hundred medical articles, eighty-six teaching texts, fifty-two domestic health guides, hundreds of records from the New England Hospital for Women and Children over the course of twenty-eight years, and the personal papers of twenty-six women.
6. See, for example, Rosanne Cecil, "An Insignificant Event? Literary and Anthropological Perspectives on Pregnancy Loss," *The Anthropology of*

Pregnancy Loss: Comparative Studies in Miscarriage, Stillbirth, and Neonatal Death, ed. Rosanne Cecil (Oxford: Berg, 1996), 1–14; Patricia Jeffery and Roger Jeffery, "Delayed Periods and Falling Babies: The Ethnophysiology and Politics of Pregnancy Loss in Rural North India," in *The Anthropology of Pregnancy Loss*, 17–37; Leslie Reagan, "From Hazard to Blessing to Tragedy: Representations of Miscarriage in Twentieth-Century America," *Feminist Studies* 29, no. 2 (2003): 357–378; and Sara Dubow, *Ourselves Unborn: A History of the Fetus in Modern America* (Oxford: Oxford University Press, 2011).

7. Childbirth was undergoing a slow process of medicalization over the course of the nineteenth century, but by 1900 doctors still attended about only 50 percent of all births. For a history of the medicalization of childbirth, see Judith Walzer Leavitt, *Brought to Bed: Childbearing in America, 1750–1950* (Oxford: Oxford University Press, 1986).

8. Miscarriage has only recently received attention by historians of medicine, and there is still much work to be done. I am, in some sense, following in the footsteps of Leslie Reagan, who was the first historian of medicine to tackle the historical and cultural constructions of miscarriage in "From Hazard to Blessing to Tragedy: Representations of Miscarriage in Twentieth-Century America." Anthropologists and sociologists have a longer tradition of considering pregnancy loss: see Rosanne Cecil, ed., *The Anthropology of Pregnancy Loss*; and Linda Layne, *Motherhood Lost: A Feminist Account of Pregnancy Loss in America* (New York: Routledge, 2003).

9. The history of reproduction is vast and cited throughout this book. One helpful overview is Leslie J. Reagan's "Medicine, Law, and the State: The History of Reproduction," *Companion to American Women's History*, ed. Nancy A. Hewitt (New York: Blackwell Publishers, 2002), 348–365.

10. For more on the early twentieth-century hunt for embryos, see Lynn M. Morgan, *Icons of Life: A Cultural History of Human Embryos* (Berkeley: University of California Press, 2009); and Sara Dubow, *Ourselves Unborn*.

11. Edwin M. Hale, *A Systematic Treatise on Abortion* (Chicago: C. S. Halsey, 1866), xiii.

12. To give just one example, in 1828 Dr. James Blundell described "the placenta of a full-grown ovum of nine months" in "On the Earlier and

Later Floodings," *Boston Medical and Surgical Journal* 1, no. 38 (1828): 612–618, quotation on 615.

13. Sociologist Linda Layne was perhaps the first scholar to address this theme with "Breaking the Silence: An Agenda for a Feminist Discourse of Pregnancy Loss," *Feminist Studies* 23, no. 2 (1997): 289–315. Medical researchers have also recently begun to study this phenomenon; see Johan Bardos, Daneil Hercz, Jenna Friedenthal, Stacey Missmer, and Zev Williams, "A National Survey on Public Perceptions of Miscarriage," *Obstetrics and Gynecology* 125, no. 6 (2015): 1313–1320. This call to action has become more mainstream (if perhaps still not answered) in recent years with, for example, Lynn Snowden Pickett, "Breaking the Silence about Miscarriage," *Self* 27, no. 4 (April 1, 2005); or Lara Freidenfelds, "Yes, We Should Tell about Our Miscarriages on Facebook," *Nursing Clio* (August 28, 2015), https://nursingclio.org/2015/08/18/yes-we-should-tell-about-our-miscarriages-on-facebook/.

14. See, for example, X. Wang, C. Chen, L. Wang, D. Chen, W. Guang, and J. French, "Conception, Early Pregnancy Loss, and Time to Clinical Pregnancy: A Population-Based Study," *Fertility and Sterility* 79, no. 3 (2003): 577–584.

1. Oh Joy, Oh Rapture

1. A quick Google search on "miscarriage" finds media accounts of music icon Beyoncé's miscarriage and sadness, the heartache a television actress felt in the wake of her miscarriage, and numerous responses to Facebook founder Mark Zuckerberg's post about the loneliness and grief he and his wife felt after a miscarriage.

2. Edward H. Clarke, *Sex in Education; or, A Fair Chance for Girls* (New York: Houghton, Mifflin and Company, 1873).

3. Alice Kirk Grierson, *The Colonel's Lady on the Western Frontier: The Correspondence of Alice Kirk Grierson* (Lincoln: University of Nebraska Press, 1989), 58–63.

4. For a good analysis of both available primary sources and the continuing historiographical discussion about tracking and understanding fertility rates in the United States, see Susan E. Klepp, *Revolutionary Conceptions:*

Women, Fertility, and Family Limitation in America, 1760–1820 (Chapel Hill: University of North Carolina Press, 2009).

5. Andrea Tone, *Devices and Desires: A History of Contraceptives in America* (New York: Hill and Wang, 2001); Linda Gordon, *The Moral Property of Woman: A History of Birth Control Politics in America*, 3rd ed. (Urbana: University of Illinois Press, 2002); and James Reed, *From Private Vice to Public Virtue: The Birth Control Movement and American Society since 1830* (New York: Basic Books, 1978).

6. Janet Farrell Brodie, *Contraception and Abortion in 19th-Century America* (Ithaca, N.Y.: Cornell University Press, 1994); and Tone, *Devices and Desires*.

7. James C. Mohr, *Abortion in America: The Origins and Evolutions of National Policy, 1800–1900* (New York: Oxford University Press, 1987); and Leslie Reagan, *When Abortion Was a Crime: Women, Medicine, and Law in the United States, 1867–1973* (Berkeley: University of California Press, 1997).

8. This was by no means a new trend; the fertility rate had been falling for almost a century by then, as detailed by Klepp in *Revolutionary Conceptions*.

9. Examples include Carroll Smith-Rosenberg and Charles Rosenberg, "The Female Animal: Medical and Biological Views of Woman and Her Role in Nineteenth-Century America," *Journal of American History* 60 (1973): 332–356; Steven Mintz and Susan Kellogg, *Domestic Revolutions: A Social History of the American Family* (New York: Free Press, 1988); Nancy Cott, *The Bonds of Womanhood: "Woman's Sphere" in New England, 1780–1835* (New Haven, Conn.: Yale University Press, 1977); and John D'Emilio and Estelle B. Freedman, *Intimate Matters: A History of Sexuality in America* (New York: Harper & Row, 1988).

10. See Margaret S. Marsh and Wanda Ronner, *The Empty Cradle: Infertility in America from Colonial Times to the Present* (Baltimore: Johns Hopkins University Press, 1996); and Elaine Tyler May, *Barren in the Promised Land: Childless Americans and the Pursuit of Happiness* (New York: Basic Books, 1995).

11. "Being sick" was a common nineteenth-century euphemism for childbirth.

12. Emily McCorkle FitzGerald, *An Army Doctor's Wife on the Frontier: Letters from Alaska and the Far West, 1874–1878*, ed. Abe Laufe (Pittsburgh, Pa.: University of Pittsburgh Press, 1962), 5–66.

13. Ibid., 165.

14. Ibid.

15. Indeed, the rhythm method was perhaps popular with many women, who had limited access to or personal conflicts with other methods of birth control. See "A Story of Love and Family Limitation: 'x' for Sexual Intercourse," in Brodie's *Contraception and Abortion in 19th-Century America*, 9–37.

16. FitzGerald, *An Army Doctor's Wife on the Frontier*, 165.

17. I have presented Annie Youmans Van Ness's writings as she did, complete with grammatical and spelling errors. Her entries are frequently devoid of commas or periods, which often caused me to imagine her speaking at a breakneck pace.

18. Annie L. Youmans Van Ness, *Diary of Annie L. Van Ness, 1864–1881* (Alexandria, Va.: Alexander Street Press, 2004), 3 and 637.

19. Ibid., 639 and 651.

20. Ibid., 629, 663, 681, and 684.

21. Ibid., 685.

22. William Edward Buckley, *A New England Pattern: The History of Manchester, Connecticut* (Chester, Conn.: Pequot Press, 1973), 88–91.

23. Mary Bushnell Cheney, letter to Frank Cheney, June 24, 1879, Cheney Family Papers, box 1, folder 1, Sophia Smith Collection, Smith College, Northampton, Mass.

24. I would like to thank the anonymous reviewer who pointed out that Cheney's happy exclamation probably derived from a familiarity with the Gilbert and Sullivan musical *H.M.S. Pinafore* whose finale is titled "Oh joy, oh rapture unforeseen." The musical was very popular on the East Coast in 1878 and 1879, indicating that even if Cheney did not see the musical herself, she was likely very aware of it and its music. John Bush Jones, *Our Musicals, Ourselves: A Social History of the American Musical Theater* (Lebanon, N.H.: Brandeis University Press, 2003), 4–7.

25. Cheney, letter to Frank Cheney, July 9, 1879, Cheney Family Papers, box 1, folder 1, Sophia Smith Collection.

26. See Janet Farrell Brodie "Menstrual Interventions in the Nineteenth-Century United States," in *Regulating Menstruation: Beliefs, Practices, Interpretations*, ed. Etienne Van De Walle and Elisha P. Renne (Chicago: University of Chicago Press, 2001), 39–63.

27. For discussions of the ambiguity between pregnancy and delayed menstruation, see Susan Klepp, "Colds, Worms, and Hysteria: Menstrual Regulation in Eighteenth-Century America," in *Regulating Menstruation*, 22–38.

28. Ella Gertrude Clanton Thomas, *The Secret Eye: The Journal of Ella Gertrude Clanton Thomas, 1848–1889*, ed. Virginia Ingraham Burr (Chapel Hill: University of North Carolina Press, 1990), 3–20. For further exploration of Thomas and other Southern women and how their lives were affected by the Civil War, see Laura Edwards, *Scarlett Doesn't Live Here Anymore: Southern Women in the Civil War Era* (Urbana: University of Illinois Press, 2000).

29. Thomas, *The Secret Eye*, 130.

30. Ibid., 148–150.

31. Ibid., 154.

32. Ibid., 212 and 254.

33. Ibid. 148.

34. Lucy McKim Garrison, letter to Ellen Wright Garrison, December 27, 1866, Garrison Family Papers, box 49, folder 17, Sophia Smith Collection, Smith College, Northampton, Mass.

35. Garrison Family Tree, created by James W. Gould, 1963, Sophia Smith Collections, http://www.smith.edu/libraries/libs/ssc/atg/popupgarrisontree.html, accessed September 21, 2013.

36. Thomas, *The Secret Eye*, 125, 135, and 212.

37. Ellen Wright Garrison, letter to Eliza Wright Osborne, August 25, 1879, Garrison Family Papers, box 36, folder 18, Sophia Smith Collection.

38. See, for example, Diary of Alice Bodman, 1883, Bodman Family Papers, box 5, folder 129, Sophia Smith Collection, Smith College, Northampton, Mass.; and Rachel Cormany, *The Cormany Diaries: A Northern Family in the Civil War*, ed. James C. Mohr and Richard Elliott Winslow (Pittsburgh, Pa.: University of Pittsburgh Press, 1982).

39. Elizabeth Cabot, Diaries, 1859–1906, entry of April 11, 1865, 81-M269-82-M14, Schlesinger Library, Radcliffe College, Cambridge, Mass.

40. Grierson, *The Colonel's Lady on the Western Frontier*, 29. Awaiting or expecting a young or little "stranger" was a common phrasing for pregnancy by this time. See Klepp, *Revolutionary Conceptions*, 109.

41. Grierson, *The Colonel's Lady on the Western Frontier*, 62–63.

42. Mary Richardson Walker, *On to Oregon: The Diaries of Mary Walker and Myra Eells*, ed. Clifford Merrill Drury (Lincoln: University of Nebraska Press, 1998), 103 and 84.

43. Blanche Butler Ames, letter to Adelbert Ames, May 12, 1871, Ames Family Papers, Sophia Smith Collection, Smith College, Northampton, Mass.

44. Ames, letter to Adelbert Ames, July 1874, Ames Family Papers, Sophia Smith Collection, emphasis in original.

45. Lucy McKim Garrison, letter to Ellen Wright Garrison, November 8, 1874, Garrison Family Papers, box 49, folder 17, Sophia Smith Collection.

46. Unfortunately, there are no children listed for her after 1873, so I cannot determine what happened with this pregnancy. Garrison herself died in 1877. See the Garrison family tree at http://www.smith.edu/libraries/libs/ssc/atg/popupgarrisontree.html.

47. Ellen Wright Garrison, letter to Eliza Wright Osborne, February 26, 1880, Garrison Family Papers, box 45, folders 4–32, Sophia Smith Collection.

48. Katherine Norton, letter to Agnes Garrison, September 19, 1898, Garrison Family Papers, Sophia Smith Collection.

49. Monica J. Casper, *The Making of the Unborn Patient: A Social Anatomy of Fetal Surgery* (New Brunswick, N.J.: Rutgers University Press, 1998), 73–105; Linda Layne, *Motherhood Lost: A Feminist Account of Pregnancy Loss in America* (New York: Routledge, 2003), 88–90; Karen Newman, *Fetal Positions: Individualism, Science, Visuality* (Stanford, Calif.: Stanford University Press, 1996), 10–18; and Barbara Katz Rothman, "Laboring Now: Current Cultural Constructions of Pregnancy, Birth, and Mothering," in *Laboring On: Birth in Transition in the United States*, ed. Wendy Simonds, Barbara Katz Rothman, and Bari Meltzer Norman (New York: Routledge, 2007), 49–52.

50. Lennart Nilsson, "Drama of Life Before Birth," *Life*, April 30, 1965, 54–65. For more about Nilsson's photographs and their effects on pregnancy thinking, see Barbara Duden, *Disembodying Women: Perspectives on Pregnancy and the Unborn* (Cambridge, Mass.: Harvard University Press, 1993), 11–24; and Rosalind Pollack Petchesky, "Fetal Images: The

Power of Visual Culture in the Politics of Reproduction," in *Reproductive Technologies: Gender, Motherhood, and Medicine*, ed. Michelle Stanworth (Minneapolis: University of Minnesota Press, 1987), 57–80.

51. Sara Dubow also critiques this link between new visualization and fetal meanings, or what she refers to as "overemphasizing the causal role of technology," in *Ourselves Unborn: A History of the Fetus in Modern America* (Oxford: Oxford University Press, 2011), 6.

52. Ames, letter to Adelbert Ames, May 12, 1871, Ames Family Papers, Sophia Smith Collection.

53. Seth Pancoast, *The Ladies' Medical Guide: A Complete Instructor and Counselor* (Philadelphia: Hubbard Bros., 1875), 257–258.

54. See, for example, Mark Jackson, "'Something More than Blood': Conflicting Accounts of Pregnancy Loss in Eighteenth-Century England," in *The Anthropology of Pregnancy Loss: Comparative Studies in Miscarriage, Stillbirth, and Neonatal Death*, ed. Rosanne Cecil (Oxford: Berg, 1996), 197–214; and Cathy McClive, "The Hidden Truth of the Belly: The Uncertainties of Pregnancy in Early Modern Europe," *Social History of Medicine* 15, no. 2 (2002): 209–227.

2. Enveloped in Mystery

1. Abigail Adams, letter to John Adams, July 9, 1777, Adams Family Papers, Massachusetts Historical Society, Boston, Mass.

2. Abigail Adams, letter to John Adams, July 10–22, 1777, Adams Family Papers, Massachusetts Historical Society.

3. Abigail Adams, letter to John Adams, July 16, 1777, Adams Family Papers, Massachusetts Historical Society.

4. This chapter relies upon writings of both European and American physicians and medical experts. In the eighteenth century, the United States was still a young country with an especially undeveloped medical profession. Texts originating in the United States were rare, and most American physicians relied upon studies and lessons coming out of European publications. Thus, the use of primarily British, Scottish, and French medical texts can still inform us of prevailing medical ideas in the United States. See Paul Starr, *The Social Transformation of American Medicine* (New York: Basic Books, 1982), 30–59.

5. Johann Storch, *Von Weiberkrankheiten, 4. Banes, I. Teil, darinnen vorne-hmlich solche Zufälle, welche Molas oder Muttergewächse und falsche Früchte betreffen* (Gotha, 1749).

6. Barbara Duden, *Disembodying Women: Perspectives on Pregnancy and the Unborn* (Cambridge, Mass.: Harvard University Press, 1993), 62–63.

7. Barbara Duden, "The Fetus on the 'Farther Shore': Toward a History of the Unborn," in *Fetal Subjects, Feminist Positions*, ed. Lynn M. Morgan and Meredith W. Michaels (Philadelphia: University of Pennsylvania Press, 1999), 13.

8. Cathy McClive, "The Hidden Truths of the Belly: The Uncertainties of Pregnancy in Early Modern Europe," *Social History of Medicine* 15, no. 2 (2002): 209–227.

9. Brudenell Exton, *A New and General System of Midwifery* (London: W. Owen, 1751), 16, 144.

10. Seguin Henry Jackson, *Cautions to Women, Respecting the State of Pregnancy* (London: G. G. and J. Robinson, and J. Robson, 1798), 124; Thomas Denman, *An Introduction to the Practice of Midwifery* (Vermont: William Fessenden, 1807), 58.

11. Nina Rattner Gelbart, *The King's Midwife: A History and Mystery of Madame Du Coudray* (Berkeley: University of California Press, 1998), 68.

12. McClive, "The Hidden Truths of the Belly," 215.

13. Barbara Duden, "Quick with Child: An Experience That Has Lost Its Status," *Technology in Society* 14 (1992): 335–344, on p. 336.

14. McClive, "The Hidden Truths of the Belly," 215–220.

15. See, for example, Clara Pinto-Correia, *Ovary of Eve: Egg and Sperm and Preformation* (Chicago: University of Chicago Press, 1997).

16. Pinto-Correia, *Ovary of Eve*, xv.

17. Shirley A. Roe, *Matter, Life, and Generation: Eighteenth-Century Embryology and the Haller-Wolff Debate* (Cambridge: Cambridge University Press, 1981); Peter Hanns Reill, *Vitalizing Nature in the Enlightenment* (Berkeley: University of California Press, 2005); and Nick Hopwood, "Embryology," in *The Cambridge History of Science*, Volume 6: *The Modern Biological and Earth Sciences*, ed. Peter J. Bowler and John V. Pickstone (Cambridge: Cambridge University Press, 2009), 285–315.

18. François Mauriceau, *The Diseases of Women with Child*, trans. Hugh Chamberlen (London, 1727), 10.

19. Ibid., 26–27.

20. Ibid., 118.

21. Pierre Dionis, *A General Treatise of Midwifery* (London: A. Bell, 1719), 145.

22. Mark Jackson, "'Something More than Blood': Conflicting Accounts of Pregnancy Loss in Eighteenth-Century England," in *The Anthropology of Pregnancy Loss: Comparative Studies in Miscarriage, Stillbirth, and Neonatal Death*, ed. Rosanne Cecil (Oxford: Berg, 1996), 197–214. For more on the slippage between menstruation, pregnancy, illness, and abortion, and the concept of "bringing on the menses," see Janet Farrell Brodie, "Menstrual Interventions in the Nineteenth-Century United States," and Gigi Santow, "Emmenagogues and Abortifacients in the Twentieth Century: An Issue of Ambiguity," both in *Regulating Menstruation: Beliefs, Practices, Interpretations*, ed. Etienne Van De Walle and Elisha P. Renne (Chicago: University of Chicago Press, 2001).

23. Monica Helen Green, "From 'Diseases of Women' to 'Secrets of Women': The Transformation of Gynecological Literature in the Later Middle Ages," *Journal of Medieval and Early Modern Studies* 30, no. 1 (2000): 5–39.

24. Katharine Park, *Secrets of Women: Gender, Generation, and the Origins of Human Dissection* (New York: Zone Books, 2006), 77–120.

25. Fielding Ould, *A Treatise of Midwifery* (London, 1748), 137–138.

26. Mary Coke, *The Letters and Journals of Lady Mary Coke*, ed. James Archibald Home (Bath: Kingsmead Bookshops, 1970), 221.

27. Ibid., 331, 446.

28. Mary Clavering Cowper, *Diary of Mary Countess Cowper, Lady of the Bedchamber to the Princess of Wales, 1714–1720* (London: J. Murray, 1865), 46, 105.

29. Linda A. Pollock, "Embarking on a Rough Passage: The Experience of Pregnancy in Early-Modern Society," in *Women as Mothers in Pre-Industrial England*, ed. Valerie Fildes (New York: Routledge, 1990), 39–67. See also Laura Gowing, *Common Bodies: Women, Touch, and Power in Seventeenth-Century England* (New Haven, Conn.: Yale University Press, 2003).

30. Samuel Bard, *A Compendium of the Theory and Practice of Midwifery* (New York: Collins and Co., 1819), 365.

31. Sandee Hathaway, Arlene Eisenberg, Heidi Murkoff, and Sharon Mazel, *What to Expect When You're Expecting, 4th Edition* (New York: Workman Publishing Co., 2008).

32. William Buchan, *Domestic Medicine* (Philadelphia, 1774), 397. Paul Starr claims that this book was the most influential of its kind, published originally in Edinburgh in 1769, and in Philadelphia only two years later. Starr, *The Social Transformation of American Medicine*, 32–33.

33. Starr, *The Social Transformation of American Medicine*, 30–59.

34. James Spear Loring, *The Hundred Boston Orators Appointed by the Municipal Authorities and Other Public Bodies from 1770 to 1852* (Boston: John P. Jewett & Co., 1855), 482.

35. Lucretia Peabody Everett letter to Sarah Everett Hale, August 9, 1820, box 110, folder 23, Hale Family Papers, Sophia Smith Collection, Smith College, Northampton, Mass.

36. Ibid., underlining in original.

37. Everett, letter to Hale, March 20, 1823, Hale Family Papers, Sophia Smith Collection, underlining in original.

38. Ibid.

39. Judith Walzer Leavitt, *Brought to Bed: Childbearing in America, 1750–1950* (New York: Oxford University Press, 1986), 36–63.

40. For nineteenth-century birthing trends, see Leavitt, *Brought to Bed*, 12.

3. Before Its Due Time

1. Amelia Ryerse Harris, *The Eldon House Diaries: Five Women's Views of the 19th Century*, ed. Robin Sutton Harris and Terry G. Harris (Toronto: Champlain Society, 1994), 255.

2. Ibid.

3. Thomas Denman, *An Introduction to the Practice of Midwifery* (Brattleborough, Vt.: William Fessenden, 1807), 58.

4. Aristotle, *On the Generation of Animals*, Book II, trans. Arthur Platt (eBooks@Adelaide 2007), 1, https://ebooks.adelaide.edu.au/a/aristotle/generation/book2.html. Linda Van Speygroeck, Dani De Waele, and Gertrudis Ven De Vijver, "Theories in Early Embryology: Close Connections between Epigenesis, Preformationism, and Self-Organization," *Annals of the New York Academy of Science* 981 (2002): 7–49. See also Joseph

Needham, *A History of Embryology* (Cambridge: Cambridge University Press, 1934), 21; Jane Oppenheimer, *Essays in the History of Embryology and Biology* (Cambridge, Mass.: M.I.T. Press, 1967), 122; and Shirley A. Roe, *Matter, Life, and Generation: Eighteenth-Century Embryology and the Haller-Wolff Debate* (Cambridge: Cambridge University Press, 1981), 3.

5. Shirley Roe, "John Tuberville Needham and the Generation of Living Organisms," *Isis* 74, no. 2 (1983): 159–184; and Peter Hanns Reill, *Vitalizing Nature in the Enlightenment* (Berkeley: University of California Press, 2005), 159–171. Joseph Needham also claims that the Aristotelian roots of epigenesis made it unfashionable in the seventeenth century; see *A History of Embryology*, 147.

6. For a discussion of the complexities of the rise of men-midwives across multiple European countries, see *The Art of Midwifery: Early Modern Midwives in Europe*, ed. Hilary Marland (London: Routledge, 1993).

7. Reill, *Vitalizing Nature in the Enlightenment*, 165.

8. Roe, *Matter, Life, and Generation*, 150–152.

9. Frederick B. Churchill, "The Rise of Classic Descriptive Embryology," in *A Conceptual History of Modern Embryology*, ed. Scott F. Gilbert (New York: Plenum Press, 1985), 1–30.

10. Jane Maienschein, *Whose View of Life? Embryos, Cloning, and Stem Cells* (Cambridge, Mass.: Harvard University Press, 2003), 21.

11. As quoted in Alexander Keiller, "Cases of Hysteria and Spurious Pregnancy," *American Journal of the Medical Sciences* 28 (1854): 265–269.

12. Charles D. Meigs, *Obstetrics: The Science and the Art* (Philadelphia: Henry C. Lea, 1867), 247.

13. John Aitken, *Principles of Midwifery, Or Puerperal Medicine* (Edinburgh, 1784), 71.

14. However, the physician Alexander Hamilton might have been uncle to the American founding father Alexander Hamilton; see Ron Chernow, *Alexander Hamilton* (New York: Penguin Books, 2004), 13. Jean Astruc, *A Treatise on all the Diseases Incident to Women* (London: T. Cooper, 1743), 358; Alexander Hamilton, *Outlines of the Theory and Practice of Midwifery* (Edinburgh: Charles Elliot, 1787), 181.

15. François Mauriceau, *The Disease of Women With Child: As Also, the Best Means of Helping Them in Natural and Unnatural Labours*, ed. Hugh Chamberlen (R. Ware, London, 1755), 110.

16. Edwin M. Hale, *A Systematic Treatise on Abortion* (Chicago: C. S. Halsey, 1866), xiii.

17. See, for example, Fleetwood Churchill, *On the Theory and Practice of Midwifery* (Philadelphia: Blanchard and Lea, 1853); Gunning S. Bedford, *The Principles and Practice of Obstetrics* (New York: William Wood & Co., 1874); Alfred Lewis Galabin, *A Manual of Midwifery* (London: J. & A. Churchill, 1886); William Easterly Ashton, *Essentials of Obstetrics* (Philadelphia: W. B. Saunders, 1894).

18. Charles D. Meigs, *Woman: Her Diseases and Remedies* (Philadelphia: Lea and Blanchard, 1851), 539 and 546.

19. Gunning S. Bedford, *The Principles and Practice of Obstetrics*, 266.

20. See, for example, Thomas Cock, *A Manual of Obstetrics* (New York: Samuel S. & William Wood, 1853), 105; John King, *American Eclectic Obstetrics* (Cincinnati: Moore, Wilstach, Keys & Co., 1855), 67; B. L. Hill, *Illustrated Midwifery; or, Lectures on Obstetrics, and the Diseases of Women and Children* (Cincinnati: J. W. Sewell & Co., 1860), 73; and Hugh Lenox Hodge, *The Principles and Practice of Obstetrics* (Philadelphia: Blanchard and Lea, 1864), 464.

21. A. I. Cummings, "Use of the Tampon in Abortion," *Boston Medical and Surgical Journal* 49 (1854): 99. Italics in original. *Guttatim* is a medical term from the Latin word that means drop by drop.

22. John G. Holston, "Remarkable Case of Premature Labor; Embryulcia," *Medical and Surgical Reporter* 15, no. 25 (1866): 526–527; Horatio C. Wood, "Case of Miscarriage," *Medical and Surgical Reporter* 10, no. 3 (1863): 38.

23. Charles E. Rosenberg, "Health in the Home: A Tradition of Print and Practice," in *Right Living: An Anglo-American Tradition of Self-Help Medicine and Hygiene*, ed. Charles E. Rosenberg (Baltimore: Johns Hopkins University Press, 2003), 1–20; and Janet Farrell Brodie, *Contraception and Abortion in Nineteenth-Century America* (Ithaca, N.Y.: Cornell University Press, 1994).

24. Paul Starr, *The Social Transformation of American Medicine* (New York: Basic Books, 1982), 44–54.

25. For more on physiological societies as a form of medical self-reliance, see Martha H. Verbrugge, *Able-Bodied Womanhood: Personal Health and Social Change in Nineteenth-Century Boston* (New York: Oxford University Press, 1988).

26. Norman Gevitz, "Domestic Medical Guides and the Drug Trade in Nineteenth-Century America," *Pharmacy in History* 32, no. 2 (1990): 51–56.

27. Carl F. Kaestle, Helen Damon-Moore, Lawrence C. Stedman, Katherine Tinsley, and William Vance Trollinger, Jr., *Literacy in the United States: Readers and Reading since 1880* (New Haven, Conn.: Yale University Press, 1991), 247.

28. Brodie, *Contraception and Abortion in Nineteenth-Century America*, 158–159, 163.

29. Kaestle et al., *Literacy in the United States*, 248.

30. Sarah Leavitt, *From Catharine Beecher to Martha Stewart: A Cultural History of Domestic Advice* (Chapel Hill: University of North Carolina Press, 2002), 10.

31. Alfred G. Hall, *The Mother's Own Book and Practical Guide to Health* (Rochester, N.Y., 1843), 132.

32. John C. Gunn, *Gunn's New Domestic Physician: Or, Home Book of Health* (Cincinnati: Moore, Wilstach, Keys & Co., 1862), 442; P. C. Dunne, *The Young Married Lady's Private Medical Guide*, ed. and trans. A. F. Derbois and F. Harrison Doane (Boston, 1854), 261.

33. A. M. Mauriceau, *The Married Woman's Private Medical Companion* (New York: J. Trow, 1860), 168–169.

34. Brodie, *Contraception and Abortion in Nineteenth-Century America*; Helen Lefkowitz Horowitz, *Rereading Sex: Battles over Sexual Knowledge and Suppression in Nineteenth-Century America* (New York: Alfred A. Knopf, 2002).

35. William Zollickoffer, "Case of Abortion—One Foetus, with Two Placentas," *Medical Examiner* 3, no. 12 (1840): 186.

36. Thomas C. Osborne, "A Case of Abortion, the Foetus Having Been Retained Four Months after Its Death," *Western Journal of Medicine and Surgery* 5, no. 2 (1846): 98–99.

37. D. W. Davis, "Abortion, Complicated with Uterine Tumor," *Boston Medical and Surgical Journal* 39, no. 18 (1848): 362.

38. Samuel Bard, *A Compendium of the Theory and Practice of Midwifery* (New York: Collins and Co., 1819), 135.

39. Edward Rigby, *A System of Midwifery* (Philadelphia: Lea & Blanchard, 1841), 142–143.

40. Placenta previa is a condition in which the placenta grows in the lower part of the uterus and covers the opening to the cervix; dysmenorrhea refers to severe uterine pain during menstruation.

41. Phthisis is progressive wasting away, usually in connection to respiratory complaints.

42. Cock, *A Manual of Obstetrics*, 105–108.

43. Hodge, *The Principles and Practice of Obstetrics*, 460.

44. Alexander Milne, *The Principles and Practice of Midwifery* (New York: Bermingham & Company, 1884), 89–91.

45. See, for example, Theophilus Parvin, *The Science and Art of Obstetrics* (Philadelphia: Lea Brothers & Co., 1886), 465; T. Gaillard Thomas, *Abortion and Its Treatment, from the Stand-Point of Practical Experience* (New York: Appleton, 1890), 16.

46. P. Cazeaux, *A Theoretical and Practical Treatise on Midwifery, Including Diseases of Pregnancy and Parturition* (Philadelphia: Lindsay and Blakiston, 1850), 253; Churchill, *On the Theory and Practice of Midwifery*, 180; King, *American Eclectic Obstetrics*, 168; D. Berry Hart, *Manual of Gynecology* (New York: Wood, 1883), 258.

47. William Leishman, *A System of Midwifery: Including the Diseases of Pregnancy and the Puerperal State* (Philadelphia: Henry C. Lea, 1875), 369.

48. J. K. Shirk, *Female Hygiene and Female Diseases* (Lancaster, Pa.: The Lancaster Publishing Co., 1884), 35.

49. W. Tyler Smith, *The Modern Practice of Midwifery: A Course of Lectures on Obstetrics* (New York: R. M. DeWitt, 1858), 178; Bedford, *The Principles and Practice of Obstetrics*, 272; John W. Comfort, *Thomsonian Practice of Midwifery, and Treatment of Complaints Peculiar to Women and Children* (Philadelphia: A. Comfort, 1845), 21; Cazeaux, *A Theoretical and Practical Treatise on Midwifery*, 253; Churchill, *On the Theory and Practice of Midwifery*, 181; King, *American Eclectic Obstetrics*, 168; Thomas Hawkes Tanner, *On the Signs and Diseases of Pregnancy* (Philadelphia: Henry C. Lea, 1868), 221.

50. Karl Schroeder, *A Manual of Midwifery* (New York: D. Appleton and Company, 1873), 146; Parvin, *The Science and Art of Obstetrics*, 466–467.

51. See, for example, Rigby, *A System of Midwifery*, 130; Galabin, *A Manual of Midwifery*, 342; Asthon, *Essentials of Obstetrics*, 101; Richard Cooper Norris, *An American Text-Book of Obstetrics* (Philadelphia: Saunders,

1895), 266; David James Evans, *Obstetrics: A Manual for Students and Practitioners* (Philadelphia: Lea, 1900), 199.

52. Churchill, *On the Theory and Practice of Midwifery*, 198; William Smoult Playfair, *A Treatise on the Science and Practice of Midwifery* (Philadelphia: Lea Bros., 1889), 223; A. S. Church, "The Causes, Treatment, and Prevention of Abortion," *The Transactions of the New York Academy of Medicine* 1 (1874): 241–253. See also William B. Atkinson, *The Therapeutics of Gynecology and Obstetrics: Comprising the Medical, Dietetic, and Hygiene Treatment of Diseases of Women* (Philadelphia: Brinton, 1880); Norris, *An American Text-Book of Obstetrics*, 266; Galabin, *A Manual of Midwifery*, 342; Ashton, *Essentials of Obstetrics*, 101; Parvin, *The Science and Art of Obstetrics*, 470; William Alexander Newman Dorland, *A Manual of Obstetrics* (Philadelphia: Saunders, 1896), 260; Evans, *Obstetrics*, 199.

53. Tanner, *On the Signs and Diseases of Pregnancy*.

54. Rigby, *A System of Midwifery*, 126.

55. A. W. Barrows, "Case of Abortion, Occurring at the Fifth Month of Gestation—Child Born Alive," *American Journal of the Medical Sciences* 50 (1853): 380–384.

56. Wood, "Case of Miscarriage."

57. Markoe, "Death of Foetus at Fifth Month Followed by Labor at Full Term," *Medical and Surgical Reporter* 17, no. 21 (1867): 446–448.

58. J. Stolz, "Respiration and Signs of Life in a Five Months Foetus," *Medical and Surgical Reporter* 15, no. 16 (1866): 344–345.

59. James C. Mohr, *Abortion in America: The Origins and Evolutions of National Policy, 1800–1900* (New York: Oxford University Press, 1978), 206–210.

60. Pye Henry Chavasse, *Advice to a Wife on the Management of Her Own Health* (New York: John Wurtele Lovell, 1880), 153.

61. Frederick Hollick, *The Matron's Manual of Midwifery; And the Diseases of Women During Pregnancy and in Childbed* (New York: Strong, 1849), 410–415.

62. James J. Davis, *A Guide to Health: Designed for Families and Others* (New York: Oakley and Mason, 1868), 115; Anna Mary Galbraith, *The Four Epochs of Woman's Life; a Study in Hygiene* (Philadelphia: W. B. Saunders & Company, 1903), 132; W. W. Hall, *Health at Home, or Hall's Family Physician* (Hartford, Conn.: James Betts & Co., 1876), 585; Alfred M. Folger, *The Family Physician: Being a Domestic Medical Work* (Spartanburg, S.C.:

Z. D. Cottrell, 1845), 226; Edward H. Dixon, *Woman, and Her Diseases, from the Cradle to the Grave: Adapted Exclusively to Her Instruction in the Physiology of Her System and All the Diseases of Her Critical Periods* (New York: Charles H. Ring, 1848), 252; Walter C. Taylor, *A Physician's Counsels to Woman in Health and Disease* (Springfield, Mass.: W. J. Holland & Co., 1871).

63. See, for example, Folger, *The Family Physician*, 226; Hollick, *The Matron's Manual of Midwifery*, 410; Dunne, *The Young Married Lady's Private Medical Guide*, 259; Mauriceau, *The Married Woman's Private Medical Companion*, 168; Pye Henry Chavasse, *Wife and Mother; or, Information for Every Woman* (Philadelphia: H. J. Smith & Co., 1888), 126; Mary Rise Melendy, *Perfect Womanhood for Maidens—Wives—Mothers* (Chicago: Monarch Book Co., 1903), 151.

64. George Napheys, *The Physical Life of Woman: Advice to the Maiden, Wife, and Mother* (Toronto: Rose Publishing Company, 1880), 148; Melendy, *Perfect Womanhood*, 151; Galbraith, *The Four Epochs of Woman's Life; a Study in Hygiene*, 132.

65. Gunn, *Gunn's New Domestic Physician*, 442–443.

66. Folger, *The Family Physician*, 226; Bedford, *The Principles and Practice of Obstetrics*, 271; Paul Fortunas Mundé, *A Sketch of the Management of Pregnancy, Parturition and the Puerperal State, Normal and Abnormal* (Detroit, Mich.: G. S. Davis, 1887), 25; Charles W. Hayt, *Obstetrics: A Manual for Students and Practitioners* (Philadelphia: Lea Brothers & Co., 1892), 66; Edwards Reynolds, *Practical Midwifery: A Handbook of Treatment* (New York: W. Wood, 1892), 55; Albert Freeman Africanus King, *A Manual of Obstetrics* (Philadelphia: Lea Brothers & Co., 1895), 162; Sheldon Leavitt, *The Science and Art of Obstetrics* (Chicago: Halsey Bros. Co., 1901), 161.

67. Folger, *The Family Physician*, 224; O. S. Fowler, *Maternity: or, The Bearing and Nursing of Children, Including Female Education and Beauty* (New York: Fowler and Wells, 1848); Stephen Tracy, *The Mother and Her Offspring* (New York: Harper & Brothers, 1853), 48; J. H. Pulte, *Woman's Medical Guide: Containing Essays on the Physical, Moral and Educational Development of Females, and the Homeopathic Treatment of Their Diseases in All Periods of Life* (Cincinnati: Moore, Anderson, Wilstach & Keys, 1853), 148; Dunne, *The Young Married Lady's Private Medical Guide*, 260; Frederick J. Garbit, *The Woman's Medical Companion and Guide to Health* (Boston: John P. Dale & Co., 1879), 139; Wilhelmine D. Schott, *Health*

*Hints to Women, Important Information for All, and the "Danish Cure"
Explained* (New York: C. P. Somerby, 1883), 228; John D. West, *Maiden-
hood and Motherhood, or, Ten Phases of Woman's Life* (Chicago: Law, King
& Law Publishing House, 1887), 472; Chavasse, *Wife and Mother*, 126;
Napheys, *The Physical Life of Woman*, 148; Melendy, *Perfect Womanhood*, 151;
Galbraith, *The Four Epochs of Woman's Life; a Study in Hygiene*, 132; Rigby,
A System of Midwifery, 128; Cock, *A Manual of Obstetrics*, 106; King, *Amer-
ican Eclectic Obstetrics*, 169; Smith, *The Modern Practice of Midwifery*, 178;
Milne, *The Principles and Practice of Midwifery*, 91; Hayt, *Obstetrics*, 66;
Ashton, *Essentials of Obstetrics*, 99; Parvin, *The Science and Art of Obstetrics*,
466; King, *A Manual of Obstetrics*, 162; Barton Cooke Hirst, *A Textbook of
Obstetrics* (Philadelphia: Lea Bros. & Co., 1888), 303; Evans, *Obstetrics*, 196.

68. Pulte, *Woman's Medical Guide*, 235; Fowler, *Maternity*, 28–31; Bedford,
    The Principles and Practice of Obstetrics, 272; Gunn, *Gunn's New Domestic
    Physician*, 443; Schroeder, *A Manual of Midwifery*, 145; Morton Monroe
    Eaton, *A Treatise on the Medical and Surgical Diseases of Women: With
    Their Homeopathic Treatment* (New York: Boericke & Tafel, 1880),
    423; Chavasse, *Wife and Mother*, 127; Henry Bixby Hemenway,
    Healthful Womanhood and Childhood (Evanston, Ill.: V. T. Hemenway and
    Company, 1894), 133; Melendy, *Perfect Womanhood*, 151.

69. Peter J. Latz, *Manual of Health for Women: Plain Advice in Sickness and
    Health* (Chicago: J. S. Hyland, 1906), 205; Chavasse, *Wife and Mother*, 132;
    Galbraith, *The Four Epochs of Woman's Life*, 132; Hemenway, *Healthful
    Womanhood and Childhood*, 133; Napheys, *The Physical Life of Woman*, 148;
    West, *Maidenhood and Motherhood*, 471.

70. Gunn, *Gunn's New Domestic Physician*, 443.

71. Chavasse, *Wife and Mother*, 132. Emphasis in original. However, given the
    limited access American women had at the time to exit an unhappy or
    dangerous marriage, this advice might have proven very useful for some.

72. Or even between reproductive health and sexual activity. Abstinence was
    often advised for postpartum recovery. See, Leavitt, *Brought to Bed*.

73. Charles Knowlton, *Fruits of Philosophy: An Essay on the Population Question*,
    2nd ed. (London: Freethought Pub. Co., 1877).

74. Brodie, *Contraception and Abortion in Nineteenth-Century America*, 105.

75. Sylvester Graham, *Lecture to Young Men* (Providence, R.I.: Weeden
    and Cory, 1834), 25, 35. Other nineteenth-century health writers created

similar lists. See, for example, Dio Lewis, *Chastity; or, Our Secret Sins* (St. Louis, Mo.: N. D. Thompson & Co., 1874), 58.

76. William A. Alcott, *The Physiology of Marriage* (Boston: John P. Jewett & Co., 1857), 118–127.

77. For more on the various groups involved in these new sexual conversations, see Horowitz, *Rereading Sex.*

78. Melendy, *Perfect Womanhood,* 151.

79. Folger, *The Family Physician,* 226; Gunn, *Gunn's New Domestic Physician,* 443.

80. Pulte, *Woman's Medical Guide,* 235–236.

81. Folger, *The Family Physician,* 226; Pulte, *Woman's Medical Guide,* 235; Dunne, *The Young Married Lady's Private Medical Guide,* 260; Gunn, *Gunn's New Domestic Physician,* 443; Chavasse, *Wife and Mother,* 126; Napheys, *The Physical Life of Woman,* 148; Galbraith, *The Four Epochs of Woman's Life,* 132; Cock, *A Manual of Obstetrics,* 106; C. Croserio, *Homoeopathic Manual of Obstetrics: Or, A Treatise on the Aid and Art of Midwifery May Derive from Homoeopathy* (Cincinnati: Moore, Wilstach, Keys & Co., 1863), 27; King, *A Manual of Obstetrics,* 162; Bedford, *The Principles and Practice of Obstetrics,* 270; Latz, *Manual of Health for Women,* 201; Hirst, *A Textbook of Obstetrics,* 243; Parvin, *The Science and Art of Obstetrics,* 466; Albert Hamilton Hayes, *Sexual Physiology of Woman, and Her Diseases: Or, Woman, Treated of Physiologically, Pathologically, and Esthetically* (Boston: Peabody Medical Institute, 1869), 151.

82. Taylor, *A Physician's Counsels to Woman,* 169.

83. Rachel Cormany, *The Cormany Diaries: A Northern Family in the Civil War,* ed. James C. Mohr and Richard Elliot (Pittsburgh: University of Pittsburgh Press, 1982), 149.

84. Ibid., 152.

85. Alice Pratt Bodman diary, 1883–1885, Bodman Family Papers, box 5, folder 130, Sophia Smith Collection, Smith College, Northampton, Mass.

86. Blanche Butler Ames, letter to Adelbert Ames, May 12, 1871, Ames Family Papers, box 44, folder 1, Sophia Smith Collection, Smith College, Northampton, Mass.; Mina M. Hinds Diary of 1870, Mina M. Hinds Diaries, Schlesinger Library, Radcliffe College, Cambridge, Mass.

87. Elizabeth Rogers Mason Cabot, *More than Common Powers of Perception: The Diary of Elizabeth Rogers Mason Cabot,* ed. P.A.M. Taylor (Boston: Beacon Press, 1991), 252–254.

88. Emily McCorkle FitzGerald, *An Army Doctor's Wife on the Frontier: Letters from Alaska and the Far West, 1874–1878*, ed. Abe Laufe (Pittsburgh: University of Pittsburgh Press, 1962), 5–66.

89. Ames, letter to Adelbert Ames, June 25, 1871, Ames Family Papers, Sophia Smith Collection, emphasis in original. Although this lamentation may also have been a self-imposed restriction based on not going out in public during pregnancy. See Shannon Withycombe, "Unusual Fontal Developments: Negotiating the Pregnant Body in Nineteenth-Century America," *Journal of Women's History* 27, no. 4 (2015): 160–183.

90. Adelbert Ames, letter to Blanche Butler Ames, June 28, 1871, box 18, folder (4–10), Ames Family Papers, Sophia Smith Collection.

91. Ellen Wright Garrison, letter to Eliza Wright Osborne, August 25, 1879, Garrison Family Papers, box 36, folder 18, Sophia Smith Collection.

92. Katherine Garrison Norton, letter to Agnes Garrison, December 21, 1898, Garrison Family Papers, box 94, folder 1, Sophia Smith Collection.

93. Katherine Garrison Norton, letter to Agnes Garrison, September 19, 1898, Garrison Family Papers, box 94, folder 1, Sophia Smith Collection.

94. Dolly Lunt Burge, *The Diary of Dolly Lunt Burge, 1848–1879*, ed. Christine Jacobson Carter, (Athens, Ga.: University of Georgia Press, 1997), xxi–xxvi

95. Burge, *The Diary of Dolly Lunt Burge*, 62.

96. Tanner, *On the Signs and Diseases of Pregnancy*, 221.

97. Rosenberg, "Health in the Home," in *Right Living*, 7.

98. James Ewell, *The Medical Companion, of Family Physician: Treating Diseases of the United States*, 6th ed. (Baltimore, 1822), 484–488.

99. John C. Gunn, *Gunn's Domestic Medicine, or Poor Man's Friend* (Knoxville, Tenn.: F. S. Heiskell, 1833), 292–296. Bard, *A Compendium of the Theory and Practice of Midwifery*.

100. Dixon, *Woman, and Her Diseases*, 262–263.

101. Ella Gertrude Clanton Thomas, *The Secret Eye: The Journal of Ella Gertrude Clanton Thomas, 1848–1889*, ed. Virginia Ingraham Burr (Chapel Hill: University of North Carolina Press, 1990), 148

102. Ibid., 149–150.

103. Ibid., 153.

104. Meigs, *Woman: Her Diseases and Remedies*, 27.

4. Dr. Taylor Went Up in the Uterus

1. Susan Shelby Magoffin, *Down the Santa Fe Trail and into Mexico*, ed. Stella M. Drumm (Lincoln: University of Nebraska Press, 1962), 1.

2. Ibid., 64.

3. Ibid., 66.

4. Throughout the nineteenth century, both doctors and families used the term "abortion" to refer to an accidental termination of pregnancy.

5. Magoffin, *Down the Santa Fe Trail*, 67, emphasis in original.

6. Ibid., xxxii.

7. Stuart M. Blumin, *The Emergence of the Middle Class: Social Experience in the American City, 1760–1900* (New York: Cambridge University Press, 1989).

8. Michael Haines, "Fertility and Mortality in the United States," EH.Net Encyclopedia, ed. Robert Whapels, March 19, 2008, eh.net/encyclopedia /fertility-and-mortality-in-the-united-states/.

9. For more on the development of hospitals in nineteenth- and twentieth-century America, see Charles Rosenberg, *The Care of Strangers: The Rise of America's Hospital System* (New York: Basic Books, 1987).

10. Judith Walzer Leavitt, *Brought to Bed: Childbearing in America, 1750–1950* (New York: Oxford University Press, 1986), 171–195.

11. Leavitt, *Brought to Bed*, 12.

12. Miriam Rich, "The Curse of the Civilised Woman: Race, Gender and the Pain of Childbirth in Nineteenth-Century American Medicine," *Gender and History* 28, no. 1 (April 2016): 57–76.

13. George Engelmann, "Pregnancy, Parturition, and Childbed among Primitive People," *American Journal of Obstetrics and Diseases of Women and Children* 15 (1881): 602–618.

14. P. Claiborne Gooch, "A Case of Premature Labor," *Ohio Medical and Surgical Journal* 4, no. 4 (1852): 303–304.

15. G. S. Palmer, "A Singular Case of Miscarriage and Retained Placenta," *Boston Medical and Surgical Journal* 55 (1856–1857): 445.

16. Ibid.

17. John King, *American Eclectic Obstetrics* (Cincinnati: Moore, Wilstach, Keys & Co., 1855), 177.

18. Edward Rigby, *A System of Midwifery* (Philadelphia: Lea and Blanchard, 1851), 346; Alva Curtis, *Lectures on Midwifery: And the Forms of Disease Particular to Women and Children* (Cincinnati: C. Nagel, 1846), 364.

19. John C. Pearson, "Retained Placetae in Abortion," *Medical and Surgical Reporter* 19, no. 11 (1868): 219.

20. J. T. Young, "Twin Pregnancy and Double Abortion, with Secondary Hemorrhage," *American Journal of the Medical Sciences* 56 (1868): 435.

21. L. G. Harley, "Abortion and Retained Placenta," *Medical and Surgical Reporter* 20, no. 6 (1869): 117–118. See also G. S. Palmer, "A Singular Case of Miscarriage and Retained Placenta," *Boston Medical and Surgical Journal* 55 (1856): 445.

22. Leavitt, *Brought to Bed*, 74–75.

23. Regina Markell Morantz-Sanchez, *Sympathy and Science: Women Physicians in American Medicine* (New York: Oxford University Press, 1985), 92.

24. Morantz-Sanchez, *Sympathy and Science*; Arleen Tuchman, *Science Has No Sex: The Life of Marie Zakrzewska, M.D.* (Chapel Hill: University of North Carolina Press, 2006).

25. Marie Zakrzewska, New England Hospital for Women and Children circular, 1862, New England Hospital Records, box 1, Sophia Smith Collection, Smith College, Northampton, Mass.

26. *Annual Report of the New England Hospital for Women and Children for the Year Ending November 10, 1864*, New England Hospital Records, box 2, folder 1, Sophia Smith Collection.

27. Ibid., 10.

28. Tuchman, *Science Has No Sex*, 12–22.

29. Frank G. Slaughter, *Immortal Magyar: Semmelweis, Conqueror of Childbed Fever* (New York: Schulman, 1950); Josephine Rich, *The Doctor Who Saved Babies* (New York: J. Messner, 1961); Irvine Loudon, *The Tragedy of Childbed Fever* (Oxford: Oxford University Press, 2000).

30. Rosenberg, *The Care of Strangers*, 21–24.

31. Tuchman, *Science Has No Sex*, 163–165.

32. Maternity case records, New England Hospital for Women and Children Records, no. 68, vol. 1, 1872–1873, Francis A. Countway Library of Medicine, Harvard University, Cambridge, Mass.

33. Maternity case records, New England Hospital for Women and Children Records, no. 76, vol. 2, 1874, Countway Library.

34. New England Hospital for Women and Children Records, no. 21, vol. 17, 1889, Countway Library.

35. See, for example, New England Hospital for Women and Children Records, no. 57, vol. 19, 1891; no. 94, vol. 22, 1892; no. 13, vol. 25, 1893; no. 51, vol. 27, 1895; no. 116, vol. 33, 1898; no. 207, vol. 37, 1900, Countway Library.

36. New England Hospital for Women and Children Records, no. 61, vol. 27, 1895, Countway Library.

37. New England Hospital for Women and Children Records, no. 30, vol. 31, 1897, Countway Library.

38. This timing is for pregnancy loss, which is interesting when considering doctors were "going up in" women's bodies to turn infants or other practices in childbirth decades before this. See Leavitt, *Brought to Bed*.

39. Tuchman, 10–11.

40. New England Hospital for Women and Children Records, no. 12, vol. 12, 1884, Countway Library.

41. New England Hospital for Women and Children Records, no. 59, vol. 7, 1879; no. 11, vol. 9, 1881; and no. 21, vol. 17, 1889, Countway Library.

42. New England Hospital for Women and Children Records, no, 87, vol. 17, 1889, Countway Library.

43. J. A. Spalding, *Illustrated Popular Biography of Connecticut* (Hartford, Conn.: Case, Lockwood & Brainard Company, 1891), 306.

44. List of Births Attended by Charles E. Brayton, November 3, 1874, Rubenstein Library, Duke University, Durham, N.C.

45. Statistics compiled from the 1880 United States Census for Stonington, Connecticut.

46. List of Births Attended by Charles E. Brayton, Rubenstein Library.

47. List of Births Attended by Charles E. Brayton, January 22, 1880; July 31, 1880; March 16, 1892; June 10, 1895, Rubenstein Library.

48. *War Letters of William Thompson Lusk: Captain, Assistant Adjutant-General, United States Volunteers 1861–1863 Afterward M.D., LL.D.* (New York: 1911), 7–18.

49. "Dr. William T. Lusk of New York Obituary," *Medical News* (June 19, 1897): 837.

50. However, the lectures could also have come from Lusk's short stint as lecturer at Harvard University in 1871.

51. "Dr. William T. Lusk of New York Obituary," 837.

52. William T. Lusk, "Abortion," *Medical and Surgical Journal* 33, no. 24 (December 11, 1875): 461–465; William T. Lusk, "Abortion," *Medical and Surgical Journal* 33, no. 25 (December 18, 1875): 481–484; William T. Lusk, "Abortion," *Medical and Surgical Journal* 33, no. 26 (December 25, 1875): 501–504.

53. Lusk, "Abortion," (December 25, 1875): 504.

54. Lusk, "Abortion," (December 11, 1875): 462. The decidua is a mucous membrane that lines the uterus during pregnancy and serves as the maternal portion of the placenta.

55. Lusk, "Abortion," (December 18, 1875): 483.

56. Ibid., 484.

57. Judith Leavitt shows similar findings in the case of childbirth, although she dates it a bit earlier in the century; see Leavitt, *Brought to Bed*, 36–63.

58. Henry A. Martin, *Of Miscarriage, and Especially of the Use of Loomis's Forceps in Its Management* (Chicago: Bulletin Printing Co., 1879).

59. Henry J. Garrigues, "The Treatment of Abortion," *Medical News* 71, no. 19 (November 6, 1897): 589–592.

60. Thaddeus L. Leavitt, "Peritonitis—Abortion," *Medical and Surgical Reporter* 14, no. 26 (June 30, 1866): 501.

61. C. H. Shivers, "Retained Placenta; Removal," *Medical and Surgical Reporter* 60, no. 14 (April 6, 1889): 439–440.

62. See, for example, John G. Holston, "Remarkable Case of Premature Labor: Embryulcia," *Medical and Surgical Review* 15, no. 25 (December 22, 1866): 526–527; Horatio C. Wood, "Case of Miscarriage," *Medical and Surgical Reporter* 10, no. 3 (May 16, 1863): 38; and Eugene Cordell, "Profuse Flooding at Seventh Week of Pregnancy, with Artificial Delivery of Ovum," *Medical and Surgical Reporter* 45, no. 11 (September 10, 1881): 295.

63. See, for example, J. V. Kendall, "A Case of Tetanus after Miscarriage," *Transactions of the Medical Society of New York* (1876): 185–191; S. R. Humston, "Puerperal Convulsions after Miscarriage," *Medical and Surgical Reporter* 56, no. 17 (April 23, 1887): 541; F. M. Ganett, "A Case of

Fourteen Successive Miscarriages, Terminating in Chorea," *New York Journal of Medicine and Collateral Sciences* 13, no. 2 (September, 1854): 238–239.

64. A. I. Cummings, "Use of the Tampon in Abortion," *Boston Medical and Surgical Journal* 49 (1854): 98–99. Italics in original.

65. "Embryonic Miscarriage," *Medical and Surgical Reporter* 77, no. 2 (1897): 53–55.

66. A. J. Swaney, "Retained Placenta in Miscarriage—How Shall We Treat Such Cases?," *Medical and Surgical Reporter* 64, no. 23 (June 6, 1891): 721–723.

67. Alexander H. P. Leuf, *Gynecology, Obstetrics, Menopause* (Philadelphia: Philadelphia Medical Council, 1902), 83. See also A. L. Clark, "How Shall We Treat Retained Placenta in Abortions?," *The Physicians' and Surgeons' Investigator* 4, no. 8 (1883): 247–249.

68. Francis Henry Davenport, *Diseases of Women; a Manual of Non-Surgical Gynecology, Designed Especially for the Use of Students and General Practitioners* (Philadelphia: Lea Brothers & Co., 1889); Henry J. Garrigues, "The Treatment of Abortion," *Medical News* 71, no. 19 (1897): 589–592; J. S. Baer, "The Treatment of Abortion, with Remarks upon the Use of Ergot," *Medical and Surgical Reporter* 77, no. 2 (1897): 39–41.

69. See, for example, Kendall, "A Case of Tetanus after Miscarriage"; Banga, "Fatal Tetanus Accompanying Retention of a Segment of the Placenta Four Weeks after Miscarriage"; James King Crook, "A Contribution to the Natural History of Pulmonary Consumption," *Medical Record* 29 (1886): 323–329.

70. T. Gaillard Thomas, *Abortion and Its Treatment, from the Stand-Point of Practical Experience* (New York: Appleton, 1890), 45; William Heath Byford, *A Treatise on the Theory and Practice of Obstetrics* (New York: W. Wood & Co., 1870), 161.

71. W. Tyler Smith, *The Modern Practice of Midwifery: A Course of Lectures on Obstetrics* (New York: R. M. DeWitt, 1858), 197.

72. Gunning S. Bedford, *The Principles and Practice of Obstetrics* (New York: Samuel S. & William Wood, 1861), 281.

73. Edward A. Spooner, "On Abortion," *Medical and Surgical Reporter* 11, no. 3 (1864): 1–3.

74. See, for example, A. R Nelson, "A Case of Abortion, and Retention of the Placenta," *Western Journal of Medicine and Surgery* 5, no. 1 (1846): 9–11.

75. Obstetrical Society of London, *Catalogue and Report of Obstetrical and Other Instruments Exhibited at the Conversazione of the Obstetrical Society of London* (London: Longmans, Green and Co., 1866), 6.

76. Ibid., 43.

77. Matthews Brothers, *A Catalogue of Surgical Instruments Manufactured and Supplied by Matthews Brothers* (London: Matthews Brothers, 1874).

78. William Hatteroth's Surgical House, *Surgical Instruments* (San Francisco: Wm. Hatteroth's Surgical House, 1899), 99.

79. Paul F. Mundé, *A Sketch of the Management of Pregnancy, Parturition and the Puerperal State, Normal and Abnormal* (Detroit, Mich.: G. S. Davis, 1887), 28.

80. Hiram Von Sweringen, "The Treatment of Retained Placenta after Abortion," *Obstetric Gazette* 6, no. 6 (1883): 294.

81. Davenport, *Diseases of Women*, 279. However, sharp curettes carried the danger of perforation of the uterine wall.

82. Evans, *Obstetrics*, 200.

83. Andrew F. Currier, "Spontaneous Expulsion of Uterine Fibro-Myomata after Miscarriage"; "Observations Upon the Treatment Which Should Follow Miscarriage," *Annals of Gynecology* 1 (1887–1888): 24; "The Treatment of Inevitable Miscarriage," *Medical and Surgical Reporter* 58, no. 14 (1888): 443–445; Edward Reynolds, *Practical Midwifery: A Handbook of Treatment* (New York: W. Wood, 1892), 57; Charles W. Hayt, *Obstetrics: A Manual for Students and Practitioners* (Philadelphia: Lea Brothers & Co., 1892), 69; John R. Hinkson, "Prosalpinx Following Miscarriage Successfully Removed," *Medical Record* 41, no. 14 (1892): 450; R. E. Skeel, "The Use of the Curette in Abortion," *Medical News* 62, no. 8 (1893): 207–208; Thomas, *Abortion and Its Treatment*, 83; William Easterly Ashton, *Essentials of Obstetrics Arranged in the Form of Questions and Answers Prepared Especially for Students of Medicine* (Philadelphia: W. B. Saunders, 1894), 103; Albert Freeman Africanus King, *A Manual of Obstetrics* (Philadelphia: Lea Brothers & Co., 1895), 167; G. Wyeth Cook, "The Treatment of Abortion," *Medical and Surgical Reporter* 72, no. 4 (1895): 146; George C. Barton "The Management of Miscarriage," *Medical Times and Register* 31, no. 6 (1896): 239–240; Garrigues, "The Treatment of Early Abortion by

the General Practitioner," *American Journal of Obstetrics and Diseases of Women and Children* 37 (1898): 603.

84. E. D. St Cyr, "A New Curette and Evacuator," *Medical Times and Register* 36, no. 3 (1898): 76.

85. Mila B. Sharp, "When Shall We Curette?," *Transactions of the Medical Society of Wisconsin* 31 (1897): 428.

86. Henry D. Fry, "The Indications and Contra-Indications for the Use of the Curette in Obstetrics Practice," *Journal of the American Medical Association* 37, no. 1 (1901): 617–619.

87. New England Hospital for Women and Children Records, no. 61, vol. 27, May 29, 1895, Countway Library.

88. New England Hospital for Women and Children Records, no. 44, vol. 28, September 23, 1895, Countway Library.

89. These numbers were compiled from examining every record in the maternity ward and indicate all who self-reported a previous miscarriage.

90. J. A. Baughman, "Miscarriage Produced by Gunshot Wound Penetrating the Uterus," *Journal of the American Medical Association* 28, no. 9 (February 27, 1897): 406–407.

91. New England Hospital for Women and Children Records, no. 36, vol. 28, 1895, Countway Library.

5. The Body in the Clot

1. Caroline Healey Dall, *Daughter of Boston: The Extraordinary Diary of a Nineteenth-Century Woman* (Boston: Beacon Press, 2005), 90–91.

2. Ibid., 102.

3. Ibid., 103.

4. Luther S. Harvey, "Exhibition of Specimens, Detroit Medical and Library Association," *Physician and Surgeon* 17, no. 3 (1895): 118.

5. Quoted in Nick Hopwood, "Producing Development: The Anatomy of Human Embryos and the Norms of Wilhelm His," *Bulletin of the History of Medicine* 74, no. 1 (2000): 35.

6. Sara Dubow examines many of these sites throughout the course of the twentieth century in *Ourselves Unborn: A History of the Fetus in Modern America* (Oxford: Oxford University Press, 2011).

7. Throughout the chapter, I use the term "embryology" to primarily indicate human embryology.

8. For further discussion of the production of scientific knowledge as a "community project" and the links between this professional knowledge and embodied social experiences, see Susan Lindee, *Moments of Truth in Genetic Medicine* (Baltimore: Johns Hopkins University Press, 2005). For another example of the coproduction of knowledge by women and doctors, see Leslie J. Reagan, *Dangerous Pregnancies: Mothers, Disabilities, and Abortion in America* (Berkeley: University of California Press, 2009).

9. See, for example, Lynn M. Morgan, *Icons of Life: A Cultural History of Human Embryos* (Berkeley: University of California Press, 2009); Jane Maienschein, *Whose View of Life? Embryos, Cloning, and Stem Cells* (Cambridge, Mass.: Harvard University Press, 2003); and Adele Clarke, *Disciplining Reproduction: Modernity, American Life Sciences, and the Problems of Sex* (Berkeley: University of California Press, 1998).

10. Ronan O'Rahilly, "One Hundred Years of Human Embryology," *Issues and Reviews in Teratology* 4 (1988): 81–128.

11. I am indebted to Leslie Reagan for the idea of the women "embedded" within scientific discoveries. This word perfectly conveys the hidden nature, and yet integral contribution, of the lay women who were often involved in reproductive science. See *Dangerous Pregnancies.*

12. For a discussion of Wilhelm His's disdain for physicians, see Nick Hopwood, "Producing Development."

13. Analysis of embryology and social meanings of the fetus is scant for the nineteenth century. For early twentieth-century analysis, see Sara Dubow, *Ourselves Unborn*; and Lynn M. Morgan, *Icons of Life.*

14. Nick Hopwood mentions the importance of this first step in German embryo collecting as well in "Producing Development," 38–39.

15. Judith Leavitt shows us that in 1850 almost all American births took place in the home, and by 1900, that number had only dropped to around 80 percent. Leavitt, *Brought to Bed: Childbearing in America, 1750 to 1950* (New York: Oxford University Press, 1986), 12.

16. Samuel Bard, *A Compendium of the Theory and Practice of Midwifery* (New York: Collins and Co., 1819), 54.

17. William Potts Dewees, *A Compendious System of Midwifery* (Philadelphia: Carey and Lea, 1832), 89.

18. Nick Hopwood presents another way to think of the results of the shift from preformation to epigenesis: "Earlier naturalists had represented external surfaces; anatomists now dissected organisms to reveal the inner structural relations and functional activities of the parts"; see Hopwood, "Embryology," in *The Cambridge History of Science*, Volume 6: *The Modern Biological and Earth Sciences*, ed. Peter J. Bowler and John V. Pickstone (Cambridge: Cambridge University Press, 2009), 285–315, quotation on 287–288.

19. A. Lopez, "Account of a Blighted Foetus of the Third Month, Having the Umbilicus Cord Extensively Coiled Around the Right Knee and Lower Third of Thigh, Discharged with a Living Child at Full Term," *American Journal of the Medical Sciences* 24 (1846): 309–330.

20. Ibid.

21. Henry Miller, *The Principles and Practice of Obstetrics* (Philadelphia: Blanchard and Lea, 1858), 118–167. The decidua is the membrane that lines the uterus during pregnancy.

22. E. Chenery, "A Case of Double Conception Bearing on the Question of Superfoetation," *Boston Medical and Surgical Journal* 7, no. 15 (1871): 242.

23. Nick Hopwood and Jane Maienschein also contend that abortion and miscarriage accounted for most of the human embryological specimens. See Hopwood, "Producing Development," 38; and Maienschein, *Whose View of Life?*, 63.

24. "St. Louis Medical Society," *Weekly Medical Review*, 9 (1884): 294–298.

25. Alex Y. P. Garnett, "Abnormal Adhesion of Funis to Placenta, with Accidental Hemorrhage and Abortion," *American Journal of the Medical Sciences* 79, no. 157 (1880): 73–79.

26. T. R. Rubush, "Superfoetation," *Transactions of the Indiana State Medical Society* 43 (1892): 181–187.

27. James Pearson Irvine, "Second Impregnation at the Fourth Month of Utero-Gestation," *Cincinnati Lancet and Observer* 20, no. 4 (1859): 262–263.

28. Atchison, "Case of Twins at Different Stages of Development Expelled at the Same Time," *American Journal of the Medical Sciences* 56 (1868): 285–286.

29. Zollickoffer, "Case of Abortion—One Foetus, with Two Placentas," *Medical Examiner* 3, no. 12 (1840): 185–186.

30. Dall, *Daughter of Boston*, 103.

31. See, for example, Lynn M. Morgan, "'Properly Disposed of': A History of Embryo Disposal and the Changing Claims on Fetal Remains," *Medical Anthropology* 21 (2002): 247–274.

32. William C. Stevens, "Partial Abortion; Expulsion of the Amniotic Sack Alone; Three Specimens," *Transactions of the Michigan State Medical Society* 20 (1896): 609–613.

33. For discussions of the dangers of leaving miscarriage to nature, see, for example, W. A. Harvey, "Management of the Placenta in Abortion," *Boston Medical and Surgical Journal* 90 (1874): 281–283; William H. Parrish, "Some of the Bad Effects Resulting from Retained Placenta," *Philadelphia Medical Times* 12, no. 22 (1882): 743–745; and Edwin K. Ballard, "Two Cases Illustrating the Importance of Completely Emptying the Uterus Immediately after Miscarriage," *Medical News* 65, no. 11 (1894): 298–301.

34. Some examples include Leavitt, *Brought to Bed*; James C. Mohr, *Abortion in America: The Origins and Evolutions of National Policy, 1800–1900* (New York: Oxford University Press, 1978); and Linda Gordon, *The Moral Property of Women: A History of Birth Control Politics in America* (Urbana: University of Illinois Press, 2002).

35. J. H. Etheridge, "A Report of a Case of a Foetus Enclosed in Its Sister's Placenta," *Maryland Medical Journal* 13 (1885): 330–332.

36. Cephas L. Bard, "A Rare Obstetrical Case," *San Francisco Western Lancet* 1 (1872): 527–528.

37. For discussions of death in the nineteenth century, see Ann Douglas, *The Feminization of American Culture* (New York: Knopf, 1977), 200–227; Karen Halttunen, *Confidence Men and Painted Women: A Study of Middle-Class Culture in America, 1830–1870* (New Haven, Conn.: Yale University Press, 1982), 124–152; Michael Sappol, *A Traffic of Dead Bodies: Anatomy and Embodied Social Identity in Nineteenth-Century America* (Princeton, N.J.: Princeton University Press, 2002); Drew Gilpin Faust, *This Republic of Suffering: Death and the American Civil War* (New York: Alfred A. Knopf, 2008); and Gary Laderman, *The Sacred Remains: American Attitudes toward Death, 1799–1883* (New Haven, Conn.: Yale University Press, 1996).

38. See Faust, *This Republic of Suffering*.

39. Halttunen, *Confidence Men and Painted Women*; Sappol, *A Traffic of Dead Bodies*; Douglas, *The Feminization of American Culture*, 200–226.

40. J. Stolz, "Respiration and Signs of Life in a Five Months Foetus," *Medical and Surgical Reporter* 15, no. 16 (1866): 344–345.

41. Horatio Storer, *Criminal Abortion: Its Nature, Its Evidence, and Its Law* (Boston: Little, Brown, and Company, 1868), 10–11.

42. This statement is based on a survey of medical literature between 1820 and 1900, which included 86 teaching texts and over 200 articles. Storer proved ultimately successful in outlawing abortion throughout the country by the 1880s. See Mohr, *Abortion in America*.

43. S. B. Davis, "Two Foetuses of Unequal Development in the Same Uterus," *Ohio Medical and Surgical Journal* 3, no. 1 (1850): 7–10, italics in original.

44. Garnett, "Abnormal Adhesion of Funis to Placenta."

45. Laderman, *The Sacred Remains*, 9.

46. A. W. Barrows, "Case of Abortion, Occurring at the Fifth Month of Gestation—Child Born Alive," *American Journal of the Medical Sciences* 50 (1855): 308–384.

47. "Arrival of Another Distinguished Political Exile," *Water-Cure Journal* 8, no. 1 (1849): 186.

48. Charles Munde, "Water in Miscarriage," *Water-Cure Journal* 9, no. 6 (1850): 190–191, quotation on 191.

49. Victor Coste, *Histoire Générale et Particulière de Développment des Corps Organisés* (Paris, 1847).

50. James Matthews Duncan, *Researches in Obstetrics* (London, 1868), 173.

51. Thomas Hawkes Tanner, *On the Signs and Diseases of Pregnancy* (Philadelphia: Henry C. Lea, 1868), 317.

52. Duncan, *Researches in Obstetrics*, 170.

53. Gunning S. Bedford, *The Principles and Practice of Obstetrics* (New York: Wood, 1874), 442–445.

54. Tanner, *On the Signs and Diseases of Pregnancy*, 312–324; Alexander Milne, *The Principles and Practice of Midwifery* (New York: Bermingham & Company, 1884), 124–126; Bard, "A Rare Obstetrical Case"; Rodney Glisan, *Text Book of Modern Midwifery* (Philadelphia: Blakiston, 1881), 185–188; D. A. Walder, "A Case of Superfoetation," *Chicago Medical Journal and Examiner* 41, no. 1 (1880): 69–70; Samuel Nickles, "Cincinnati Academy

of Medicine," *Medical News* 47, no. 25 (1885): 690–694; Etheridge, "A Report of a Case of a Foetus Enclosed in Its Sister's Placenta"; Theophilis Parvin, *The Science and Art of Obstetrics* (Philadelphia: Lea Brothers & Co., 1886), 173–175; Matthew Darbyshire Mann, *A System of Gynecology* (Philadelphia: Lea Brothers & Co., 1887), 253; Egbert Henry Grandin, *A Text-Book of Practical Obstetrics* (Philadelphia: F. A. Davis, 1897), 181.

55. C. R. Braun, "Observations upon Superfoetation," *American Medical Times* 1 (1860): 157; George C. Hopkins, "A Case of Twin Conception: One Ovum Blighted at Three Months, and Both Carried to Full Term," *New York Medical Journal* 12, no. 2 (1870): 182–184; Bard, "A Rare Obstetrical Case"; William Goodell, "Transactions of the Philadelphia Obstetrical Society," *American Journal of Obstetrics and Diseases of Women and Children* 6, no. 2 (1873): 283–295; Achilles, "Extra-Foetation," *Cincinnati Medical News* 7, no. 6 (1878): 396–399; D. A. Walden, "A Case of Superfoetation," *Chicago Medical Journal and Examiner* 41, no. 1 (1880): 69–70; Nickles, "Cincinnati Academy of Medicine"; Etheridge, "A Report of a Case of a Foetus Enclosed in Its Sister's Placenta"; E. P. Murdock, "A Case of Superfoetation," *Chicago Medical Journal and Examiner* 57, no. 3 (September 1888): 145–146.

56. Atchinson, "Case of Twins at Different Stages of Development Expelled at the Same Time"; Chenery, "A Case of Double Conception Bearing on the Question of Superfoetation"; E. P. Allen, "Two Cases of Retained Foetus Some Months after Their Death," *Philadelphia Medical Times* 3, no. 29 (1873): 455; Rubush, "Superfoetation"; A. L. Bailey, "Superfoetation and Superfecundation with a Report of a Case of the Former," *Transactions of the Michigan Medical Society* 20 (1896): 604–608; Thomas W. Blatchford, "Blighted Foetus," *New York Journal of Medicine and Collateral Sciences* 8, no. 24 (1847): 308–312.

57. Bigelow, "A Remarkable Case of Super-Foetation," *Southern Medical and Surgical Journal* 11 (1855): 770; B. Fordyce Baker, "Case of Superfoetation," *American Medical Monthly* 4 (1855): 364–368.

58. Allen, "Two Cases of Retained Foetus Some Months After Their Death." Superfoetation is extremely rare today, and hence most of these cases were probably cases of twins in which one of the twins died.

59. Georges Louis Leclerc Buffon, *Barr's Buffon: Buffon's Natural History Containing a Theory of the Earth, a General History of Man, of the Brute Creation, and of Vegetables, Minerals, &c. &c. &c. From the French. With Notes by the Translator. In Ten Volumes* (London, 1797), 60–61.

60. Samuel Bard, *A Compendium of the Theory and Practice of Midwifery*, 53–54.

61. Thomas B. Taylor, "Case of Superfoetation and Mixed Birth," *New York Journal of Medicine* 2 (1849): 114.

62. George M. Gould and Walter L. Pyle, *Anomalies and Curiosities of Medicine* (Philadelphia: W. B. Saunders, 1900), 48.

63. Gunning S. Bedford, *The Principles and Practice of Obstetrics* (New York, 1874), 442.

64. H. E. Radisch, "Superfoetation or Superfecundation?," *Surgery, Gynecology & Obstetrics* 32, no. 4 (1921): 341.

65. I borrow this language and idea of disentangling and reentangling of embryos from Catherine Waldby and Robert Mitchell who utilize this language to argue that embryos are entangled entities in modern embryo donation programs, at times entangled in webs of kinship and at others within webs of laboratory relations. Catherine Waldby and Robert Mitchell, *Tissue Economies: Blood, Organs, and Cell Lines in Late Capitalism* (Durham, N.C.: Duke University Press, 2006), 67. Thank you to the anonymous reviewer who suggested this connection.

66. See, for example, Morgan, *Icons of Life*; Hopwood, "Producing Development"; and Clarke, *Disciplining Reproduction*.

67. Sanford B. Hunt, "Abstract of the Proceedings of the Buffalo Medical Association," *Buffalo Medical Journal* 11, no. 4 (1855): 228–233.

68. Coale, "Miscarriage; Unusual Length of the Umbilical Cord," *Boston Medical and Surgical Journal* 56 (1857): 479; Markoe, "Death of Foetus at Fifth Month Followed by Labor at Full Term," *Medical and Surgical Reporter* 17, no. 21 (1867): 446–448; Goodell, "Transactions of the Philadelphia Obstetrical Society"; Achilles, "Extra-Foetation"; Etheridge, "A Report of Case of a Foetus Enclosed in Its Sister's Placenta"; Murdock, "A Case of Superfoetation."

69. Horatio Storer, "Miscarriage from the Disease of the Foetus," *Journal of the Gynaecological Society of Boston* 5, no. 2 (1871): 77–78.

70. P. Claiborne Gooch, "A Case of Premature Labor," *Ohio Medical and Surgical Journal* 4, no. 4 (1852): 303–305.

71. Theophilus Parvin, "Macerated Fetus; Abortion Occurring in Sixth Month," *Medical and Surgical Reporter* 62, no. 15 (1890): 417–419.

72. See, for example, David James Evans, *Obstetrics: A Manual for Students and Practitioners* (Philadelphia: Lea, 1900), 196.

73. Garnett, "Abnormal Adhesion of Funis to Placenta," 175.

74. D. W. Cathell, *The Physician Himself and What He Should Add to the Strictly Scientific* (Baltimore: Cushings and Bailey, 1882), 11.

75. Stevens, "Partial Abortion."

76. Hopkins, "A Case of Twin Conception."

77. Julia Carpenter, "A Case of Miscarriage with Two Distinct Ova of Different Ages," *American Journal of Obstetrics* 20 (1887): 200–205.

78. For an excellent investigation into the program and the museum, see Shauna Devine, *Learning from the Wounded: The Civil War and the Rise of American Medical Science* (Chapel Hill: University of North Carolina Press, 2014).

79. The number reported in 1873 was 26,858, up from around 15,000 in 1871. United States Surgeon General Office, *Annual Report of the Surgeon General, United States Army* (1873), 12.

80. Joanna R. Nicholls Kyle, "The Army Medical Library and Museum," *Godey's Magazine* 136 (1898): 408–418.

81. "Cremation in a Hospital: A Dissected Fetus Burned in a Furnace," *New York Times* (1877): 12.

82. "Boys Find a Fetus," *Sioux City Journal* (1895).

83. "Another Mystery," *Los Angeles Times* (December 10, 1898): 11.

84. Lennart Nilsson, "Drama of Life Before Birth," *Life* 58, no. 17 (1965), 54–65.

85. Embryological illustrations began to appear in domestic health guides in the 1850s, with an early example being Frederick Hollick's popular *The Marriage Guide: Or, Natural History of Generation* (New York, 1850). However, these early illustrations primarily depicted late-stage pregnancies and did not focus on the developing child. In the 1870s, the imagery of embryology in popular health guides transformed, displaying earlier embryos and the alien-like forms of fetal development. See, for example, John Cowan, *The Science of a New Life* (New York: Cowan & Company,

1870), 180 and 186; and Montfort Allen and Amelia McGregor, *Glory of Woman: Or, Love, Marriage and Maternity* (Philadelphia: Elliott Publishing Co., 1896).

86. Nick Hopwood, *Embryos in Wax: Models from the Ziegler Studio* (Cambridge: Whipple Museum of the History of Science, University of Cambridge, 2002), 1.

87. Positive reactions to miscarriage should not be all that surprising, given that the history of abortion has provided many examples of nineteenth-century American women who had little desire to be pregnant. See Reagan, *When Abortion Was a Crime*; and Mohr, *Abortion in America*.

Conclusion

1. Penelope Trunk, http://twitter.com/penelopetrunk/status/4147262767, last accessed June 25, 2010.

2. "TMI" is shorthand for "too much information." Jezebel, "What Was Penelope Trunk Thinking Twittering about Her Miscarriage?," http://jezebel.com/5370535/what-was-penelope-trunk-thinking-twittering-about-her-miscarriage; ABC News, "Wisconsin Woman on Twitter: 'Thank Goodness' for Miscarriage," http://abcnews.go.com/Health/MindMoodNews/wisconsin-woman-twitters-miscarriage-loses-followers/story?id=8716315.

3. Penelope Trunk's Brazen Careerist, "You Can't Manage Your Work Life if You Can't Talk about It," http://blog.penelopetrunk.com/2009/09/24/miscarriage-is-a-workplace-event/.

4. Penelope Trunk's Brazen Careerist, "My Miscarriage—on CNN, ABC and AOL," http://blog.penelopetrunk.com/2009/10/01/my-miscarriage-on-cnn-and-aol/.

5. Penelope Trunk, "Why I Tweeted about My Miscarriage," *Guardian*, November 6, 2009, http://www.guardian.co.uk/lifeandstyle/2009/nov/06/penelope-trunk-tweet-miscarriage.

6. Mark Zuckerberg, Facebook post of July 31, 2015, https://www.facebook.com/photo.php?fbid=10102276573729791. See also Lara Freidenfelds's analysis of the post with historical context in "Yes, We Should Tell about Our Miscarriages on Facebook," Nursing Clio (blog), August 18,

2015, https://nursingclio.org/2015/08/18/yes-we-should-tell-about-our -miscarriages-on-facebook/.

7. As Rosalind Petchesky reminds us, it was a very particular historical moment that gave birth to the "the unborn," a moment that included medical authority, the allure of technology, and decades of fetal images in popular media and advertising. These factors have also helped to obscure fertility failure and diversity. Petchesky, "Fetal Images: The Power of Visual Culture in the Politics of Reproduction," *Feminist Studies* 13, no. 2 (1987): 263–292.

8. Barbara Melosh, *Strangers and Kin: The American Way of Adoption* (Cambridge, Mass.: Harvard University Press, 2002); Marie Jenkins Schwartz, *Birthing a Slave: Motherhood and Medicine in the Antebellum South* (Cambridge, Mass.: Harvard University Press, 2006).

9. Some of this work is already being done. See, for example, Ziv Eisenberg's fascinating 2013 dissertation, "The Whole Nine Months: Women, Men, and the Making of Modern Pregnancy in America" (Ph.D. diss., Harvard University, 2013).

10. See, for example, Linda Layne, *Motherhood Lost: A Feminist Account of Pregnancy Loss in America* (New York: Routledge, 2003), 88–90; Monica J. Casper, *Making of the Unborn Patient: A Social Anatomy of Fetal Surgery* (New Brunswick, N.J.: Rutgers University Press, 1998); Rosalind Petchesky, "Fetal Images: The Power of Visual Culture in the Politics of Reproduction," in *Reproductive Technologies: Gender, Motherhood, and Medicine*, ed. Michelle Stanworth (Minneapolis: University of Minnesota Press, 1987), 57–80; and Barbara Duden, *Disembodying Women: Perspectives on Pregnancy and the Unborn* (Cambridge, Mass.: Harvard University Press, 1993), 11–24.

11. These two stories are a small sample of the many experiences friends and colleagues have shared with me. Names have been changed.

12. Johan Bardos, Daniel Hercz, Jenna Friedenthal, Stacey Missmer, and Zev Williams, "A National Survey on Public Perceptions of Miscarriage," *Obstetrics and Gynecology* 125, no. 6 (2015): 1313–1320.

Index

Page numbers in *italics* indicate illustrations.

About the Author

SHANNON WITHYCOMBE is an assistant professor of history at the University of New Mexico.

Jill A. Fisher, *Medical Research for Hire: The Political Economy of Pharmaceutical Clinical Trials*

Charlene Galarneau, *Communities of Health Care Justice*

Alyshia Gálvez, *Patient Citizens, Immigrant Mothers: Mexican Women, Public Prenatal Care and the Birth Weight Paradox*

Gerald N. Grob and Howard H. Goldman, *The Dilemma of Federal Mental Health Policy: Radical Reform or Incremental Change?*

Gerald N. Grob and Allan V. Horwitz, *Diagnosis, Therapy, and Evidence: Conundrums in Modern American Medicine*

Rachel Grob, *Testing Baby: The Transformation of Newborn Screening, Parenting, and Policymaking*

Mark A. Hall and Sara Rosenbaum, eds., *The Health Care "Safety Net" in a Post-Reform World*

Laura L. Heinemann, *Transplanting Care: Shifting Commitments in Health and Care in the United States*

Laura D. Hirshbein, *American Melancholy: Constructions of Depression in the Twentieth Century*

Laura D. Hirshbein, *Smoking Privileges: Psychiatry, the Mentally Ill, and the Tobacco Industry in America*

Timothy Hoff, *Practice under Pressure: Primary Care Physicians and Their Medicine in the Twenty-first Century*

Beatrix Hoffman, Nancy Tomes, Rachel N. Grob, and Mark Schlesinger, eds., *Patients as Policy Actors*

Ruth Horowitz, *Deciding the Public Interest: Medical Licensing and Discipline*

Powel Kazanjian, *Frederick Novy and the Development of Bacteriology in American Medicine*

Rebecca M. Kluchin, *Fit to Be Tied: Sterilization and Reproductive Rights in America, 1950–1980*

Jennifer Lisa Koslow, *Cultivating Health: Los Angeles Women and Public Health Reform*

Susan C. Lawrence, *Privacy and the Past: Research, Law, Archives, Ethics*

Bonnie Lefkowitz, *Community Health Centers: A Movement and the People Who Made It Happen*

Ellen Leopold, *Under the Radar: Cancer and the Cold War*

Barbara L. Ley, *From Pink to Green: Disease Prevention and the Environmental Breast Cancer Movement*

Sonja Mackenzie, *Structural Intimacies: Sexual Stories in the Black AIDS Epidemic*

Michelle McClellan, *Lady Lushes: Gender, Alcohol, and Medicine in Modern America*

David Mechanic, *The Truth about Health Care: Why Reform Is Not Working in America*

Richard A. Meckel, *Classrooms and Clinics: Urban Schools and the Protection and Promotion of Child Health, 1870–1930*

Alyssa Picard, *Making the American Mouth: Dentists and Public Health in the Twentieth Century*

Heather Munro Prescott, *The Morning After: A History of Emergency Contraception in the United States*

Andrew R. Ruis, *Eating to Learn, Learning to Eat: School Lunches and Nutrition Policy in the United States*

James A. Schafer Jr., *The Business of Private Medical Practice: Doctors, Specialization, and Urban Change in Philadelphia, 1900–1940*

David G. Schuster, *Neurasthenic Nation: America's Search for Health, Happiness, and Comfort, 1869–1920*

Karen Seccombe and Kim A. Hoffman, *Just Don't Get Sick: Access to Health Care in the Aftermath of Welfare Reform*

Leo B. Slater, *War and Disease: Biomedical Research on Malaria in the Twentieth Century*

Paige Hall Smith, Bernice L. Hausman, and Miriam Labbok, *Beyond Health, Beyond Choice: Breastfeeding Constraints and Realities*

Matthew Smith, *An Alternative History of Hyperactivity: Food Additives and the Feingold Diet*

Susan L. Smith, *Toxic Exposures: Mustard Gas and the Health Consequences of World War II in the United States*

Rosemary A. Stevens, Charles E. Rosenberg, and Lawton R. Burns, eds., *History and Health Policy in the United States: Putting the Past Back In*

Barbra Mann Wall, *American Catholic Hospitals: A Century of Changing Markets and Missions*

Frances Ward, *The Door of Last Resort: Memoirs of a Nurse Practitioner*

Shannon Withycombe, *Lost: Miscarriage in Nineteenth-Century America*